S. Shioda, I. Homma, N. Kato (Eds.)
**Transmitters and Modulators in
Health and Disease**

S. Shioda, I. Homma, N. Kato (Eds.)

Transmitters and Modulators in Health and Disease

New Frontiers in Neuroscience

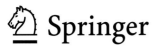

Seiji Shioda, M.D., Ph.D.
Professor
Department of Anatomy, Showa University School of Medicine
1-5-8 Hatanodai, Shinagawa-ku, Tokyo 142-8555, Japan

Ikuo Homma, M.D., Ph.D.
Professor
Department of Physiology, Showa University School of Medicine
1-5-8 Hatanodai, Shinagawa-ku, Tokyo 142-8555, Japan

Nobumasa Kato, M.D., Ph.D.
Professor
Department of Psychiatry, Karasuyama Hospital
Showa University School of Medicine
6-11-11, Kitakarasuyama, Setagaya-ku, Tokyo 157-8577, Japan

Library of Congress Control Number: 2009921985

ISBN 978-4-431-99038-3   Springer Tokyo Berlin Heidelberg New York
e-ISBN 978-4-431-99039-0

This work is subject to copyright. All rights are reserved, whether the whole or part of the material is concerned, specifically the rights of translation, reprinting, reuse of illustrations, recitation, broadcasting, reproduction on microfilms or in other ways, and storage in data banks. The use of registered names, trademarks, etc. in this publication does not imply, even in the absence of a specific statement, that such names are exempt from the relevant protective laws and regulations and therefore free for general use.
Product liability: The publisher can give no guarantee for information about drug dosage and application thereof contained in this book. In every individual case the respective user must check its accuracy by consulting other pharmaceutical literature.

Springer is a part of Springer Science+Business Media
springer.com
© Springer 2009
Printed in Japan

Typesetting: Camera-ready by the editors and authors
Printing and binding: Kato Bunmeisha, Japan

Printed on acid-free paper

Foreword

It is a great pleasure and honor to present *Transmitters and Modulators in Health and Disease*. This is a memorable scientific publication for Showa University, prepared in conjunction with the 5th International Symposium for Life Sciences, held at the university in 2008. This symposium was supported in part by Grants for the Promotion of the Advancement of Education and Research in Graduate Schools, in the program of Subsidies for Ordinary Expenses of Private Schools from the Ministry of Education, Culture, Sports, Science and Technology, Japan.

On behalf of Showa University, it is a privilege to see the publication of this volume of scientific research articles for the advancement of knowledge on brain function and morphology.

    Akiyoshi Hosoyamada, M.D., Ph.D.
    President
    Showa University, Tokyo, Japan
    January 2009

Preface

The 5th Showa International Symposium was hosted by Showa University at the university's Kamijo Auditorium on September 2, 2008. This symposium titled *Transmitters and Modulators in Health and Disease*, brought together various areas of neurosciences under a number of research themes. Six prominent researchers invited from overseas and eight speakers from Showa University gave lectures, which were followed by lively and productive discussions.

This volume includes a description of the effects of neuropeptides and biogenic amines on feeding, respiration, and other autonomic functions as well as behavior. It also considers the future use of bio-imaging tools for clinical use with patients, especially children, with neurodegenerative diseases. In the first chapter, we focus on the regulation of the blood-brain barrier function by several kinds of neuropeptides and proteins, receptors, and transporters, and in addition, on the regulatory mechanisms underlying feeding behavior and metabolism. The second chapter is concerned with the modulation of higher brain functions by neuropeptides and biogenic monoamines. Furthermore, the bio-imaging methods, using new and powerful brain-imaging techniques, also reveal human brain functions, which are presented in detail. The neuronal information processed within the brain via the auditory system and various examples of sensory information can be studied in depth with this method. The third chapter deals with the nervous system and ischemic neuronal damage by brain ischemia, as well as with hippocampal neurogenesis in the adult mouse brain. The functional significance of pro-inflammatory cytokines, pituitary adenylate cyclase-activating polypeptide (PACAP), and free radicals are also included. The results of animal experiments as well as the results of research on human tissues and organs are described. Moreover, the topic of neuroregeneration in adults, associated with regenerative medicine, is also discussed. In addition to the above-mentioned research presentations, eight poster announcements were made at the same event, generating good discussions.

The effects of employing morphological or physiological techniques to study neuropeptides and neuromodulators influencing higher-order functions or the brain stem functions, particularly of the hypothalamus, were spelled out clearly at the symposium. There was also discussion of the potential for human brain function to be investigated and for specialized medical treatment to be provided (as in the case of a vascular obstruction) by using such tools as brain navigation systems and fMRI to achieve normal higher brain function.

It would not have been possible to host the symposium without the cooperation and assistance of Showa University, for which we express our sincere gratitude.

    Seiji Shioda, M.D., Ph.D., Professor of Anatomy
    Ikuo Homma, M.D., Ph.D., Professor of Physiology
    Nobumasa Kato, M.D., Ph.D., Professor of Psychiatry
    Showa University School of Medicine
    Tokyo, Japan
    January 2009

Contents

Foreword	V
Preface	VII
Contributors	XIII
Color Plates	XXI

Neuropeptides and Behavior

Evolution of Neuropeptide Concepts Illustrated by MIF-1 and MSH
    W. Pan and A.J. Kastin 3

Increased Leptin Supply to Hypothalamus by Gene Therapy Confers Life-Long Benefits on Energy Homeostasis, Disease Cluster of Metabolic Syndrome—Diabetes Type 1 and 2, Dyslipidemia and Cardiovascular Ailments—and Bone Remodeling
    S.P. Kalra 19

Feeding Regulation in the Brain: Involvement of Neuropeptide W
    F. Takenoya, H. Kageyama, Y. Date, M. Nakazato, and S. Shioda 31

Feeding Regulation in the Brain: Role of Galanin-Like Peptide (GALP)
    H. Kageyama, F. Takenoya, and S. Shioda 41

Neuropeptides, Bioamines, and Clinical Implications

Neuropeptide Y and Its Role in Anxiety-Related Disorders
    Y. Dumont, J.C. Morales-Medina, and R. Quirion 51

The Search for a Fetal Origin for Autism: Evidence of Aberrant Brain Development in a Rat Model of Autism Produced by Prenatal Exposure to Valproate
    T. Ogawa, M. Kuwagata, and S. Shioda 83

Sexually Dimorphism and Social Brain Circuit: Its Implication to Autism
  H. Yamasue and N. Kato 89

Functional Mapping of Sensory and Motor Brain Activity

Stimulating Music: Combining Melodic Intonation Therapy with Transcranial DC Stimulation to Facilitate Speech Recovery After Stroke
  B.W. Vines, A.C. Norton, and G. Schlaug 103

Serotonin Release Acts on 5-HT2 Receptors in the Dorsomedial Medulla Oblongata to Elicit Airway Dilation in Mice
  M. Kanamaru and I. Homma 115

Breathing Is to Live, to Smell and to Feel
  Y. Masaoka and I. Homma 125

Role of the Medial Frontal Wall for Readiness of Motor Execution
  M. Inoue, Y. Masaoka, M. Kawamura, Y. Okamoto, and I. Homma 137

Poster Presentations

Ryanodine Receptor Type 1 / Calcium Release Channel in the Endoplasmic Reticulum as the Target of Nitric Oxide to Cause the Intracellular Calcium Signaling
  H. Oyamada, T. Yamazawa, T. Murayama, T. Hayashi, T. Sakurai, M. Iino, and K. Oguchi 155

Decreased Sensitivity to Negative Facial Emotions and Limbic Lesions in Patients with Myotonic Dystrophy Type 1
  M. Kawamura, A. Takeda, M. Kobayakawa, A. Suzuki, M. Kondo, and N. Tsuruya 161

Generation of Rac1 Conditional Mutant Mice by Cre/loxP System
    D. Suzuki, A. Yamada, T. Amano, A. Kimura,
    R. Yasuhara, M. Sakahara, M. Tamura, N. Tsumaki,
    S. Takeda, M. Nakamura, T. Shiroishi, A. Aiba,
    and R. Kamijo 175

Orexin Modulates Neuronal Activities of Mesencephalic Trigeminal Sensory Neurons in Rats
    K. Nakayama, A. Mochizuki, S. Nakamura,
    T. Inoue 179

Investigation of the Anxiolytic Effects of Kampo Formulation, Kamishoyosan, Used for Treating Menopausal Psychotic Syndromes in Women
    K. Toriizuka, Y. Hori, M. Fukumura, S. Isoda, Y. Hirai,
    and Y. Ida 183

Activation of Microglia Induced Learning and Memory Deficits
    S. Tanaka, H. Ohtaki, T. Nakamachi, S. Numazawa,
    S. Shioda, and T. Yoshida 191

Increased Behavioral Activity with Regular Circadian Rhythm in PACAP Specific Receptor (PAC1) Transgenic Mice
    S. Arata, T. Hosono, Y. Taketomi, H. Kageyama,
    T. Nakamachi, and S. Shioda 199

Expression and Localization of Pituitary Adenylate Cyclase-Activating Polypeptide (PACAP) Specific Receptor (PAC1R) After Traumatic Brain Injury in Mice
    K. Morikawa, K. Dohi, S. Yofu, Y. Mihara,
    T. Nakamachi, H. Ohtaki, S. Shioda, and T. Aruga 207

Key Word Index 211

Contributors

Aiba, A., Division of Molecular Biology, Department of Biochemistry and Molecular Biology, Kobe University Graduate School of Medicine, 7-5-1 Kusunoki-cho, Chuo-ku, Kobe 650-0017, Japan

Amano, T., Mouse Genomics Resource Laboratory, National Institute of Genetics, 1111 Yata, Mishima, Shizuoka 411-0801, Japan

Arata, S., Center for Biotechnology, Showa University, 1-5-8 Hatanodai, Shinagawa-ku, Tokyo 142-8555, Japan

Aruga, T., Department of Emergency and Critical Care Medicine, Showa University School of Medicine, 1-5-8 Hatanodai, Shinagawa-ku, Tokyo 142-8555, Japan

Date, Y., Department of Frontier Science Research Center, University of Miyazaki, 5200 Kiyotake, Miyazaki 889-1692, Japan

Dohi, K., Department of Emergency and Critical Care Medicine, Showa University School of Medicine, 1-5-8 Hatanodai, Shinagawa-ku, Tokyo 142-8555, Japan

Dumont, Y., Douglas Mental Health University Institute, 6875 LaSalle Boulevard, Montreal, QC, H4H 1R3, Canada

Fukumura, M., Laboratory of Pharmacognosy and Phytochemistry, School of Pharmacy, Showa University, 1-5-8 Hatanodai, Shinagawa-ku, Tokyo 142-8555, Japan

Hayashi, T., Department of Pharmacology, Showa University School of Medicine, 1-5-8 Hatanodai, Shinagawa-ku, Tokyo 142-8555, Japan

Hirai, Y., Laboratory of Herbal Garden, School of Pharmacy, Showa University, 1-5-8 Hatanodai, Shinagawa-ku, Tokyo 142-8555, Japan

Homma, I., Department of Physiology, Showa University School of Medicine, 1-5-8 Hatanodai, Shinagawa-ku, Tokyo 142-8555, Japan

Hori, Y., Laboratory of Pharmacognosy and Phytochemistry, School of Pharmacy, Showa University, 1-5-8 Hatanodai, Shinagawa-ku, Tokyo 142-8555, Japan

Hosono, T., Center for Biotechnology, Showa University, 1-5-8 Hatanodai, Shinagawa-ku, Tokyo 142-8555, Japan

Ida, Y., Laboratory of Pharmacognosy and Phytochemistry, School of Pharmacy, Showa University, 1-5-8 Hatanodai, Shinagawa-ku, Tokyo 142-8555, Japan; Yokohama College of Pharmacy, 601 Matano-cho, Totsuka-ku, Yokohama 245-0066, Japan

Iino, M., Department of Molecular Cellular Pharmacology, University of Tokyo Graduate School of Medicine, 7-3-1 Hongo, Bunkyo-ku, Tokyo 113-0033, Japan

Inoue, M., Departments of Physiology and Neurology, Showa University School of Medicine, 1-5-8 Hatanodai, Shinagawa-ku, Tokyo 142-8555, Japan

Inoue, T. Department of Oral Physiology, Showa University School of Dentistry, 1-5-8 Hatanodai, Shinagawa-ku, Tokyo 142-8555, Japan

Isoda, S., Laboratory of Herbal Garden, School of Pharmacy, Showa University, 1-5-8 Hatanodai, Shinagawa-ku, Tokyo 142-8555, Japan

Kageyama, H., Department of Anatomy, Showa University School of Medicine, 1-5-8 Hatanodai, Shinagawa-ku, Tokyo 142-8555, Japan

Kalra, S.P., Distinguished Professor, Department of Neuroscience, University of Florida College of Medicine, McKnight Brain Institute, P.O. Box 100244, Gainesville, FL 32610-0244, USA

Kamijo, R., Departments of Biochemistry, Oral Anatomy, and Developmental Biology, Showa University School of Dentistry, 1-5-8 Hatanodai, Shinagawa, Tokyo 142-8555, Japan

Kanamaru, M., Department of Physiology, Showa University School of Medicine, 1-5-8 Hatanodai, Shinagawa-ku, Tokyo 142-8555, Japan

Kastin, A.J., Blood-Brain Barrier Group, Pennington Biomedical Research Center, Baton Rouge, LA 70808, USA

Kato, **N.,** Department of Psychiatry, Showa University School of Medicine, 1-5-8 Hatanodai, Shinagawa-ku, Tokyo 142-8555, Japan

Kawamura, M., Department of Neurology, Showa University School of Medicine, 1-5-8 Hatanodai, Shinagawa-ku, Tokyo 142-8666, Japan; Core Research for Evolutional Science and Technology (CREST), Japan Science and Technology Agency (JST), Saitama, Japan

Kimura, A., Department of Orthopedic Surgery, Graduate School, Tokyo Medical and Dental University, 1-5-45 Yushima, Bunkyo-ku, Tokyo 113-8519, Japan

Kobayakawa, M., Department of Neurology, Showa University School of Medicine, 1-5-8 Hatanodai, Shinagawa-ku, Tokyo 142-8666, Japan

Kondo, M., Department of Neurology, Showa University School of Medicine, 1-5-8 Hatanodai, Shinagawa-ku, Tokyo 142-8666, Japan

Kuwagata, M., Department of Anatomy, Showa University School of Medicine, 1-5-8 Hatanodai, Shinagawa-ku, Tokyo 142-8555, Japan

Masaoka, Y., Department of Physiology, Showa University School of Medicine, 1-5-8 Hatanodai, Shinagawa-ku, Tokyo 142-8555, Japan

Mihara, Y., Department of Emergency and Critical Care Medicine, Showa University School of Medicine, 1-5-8 Hatanodai, Shinagawa-ku, Tokyo 142-8555, Japan

Mochizuki, A., Department of Oral Physiology, Showa University School of Dentistry, 1-5-8 Hatanodai, Shinagawa-ku, Tokyo 142-8555, Japan

Morales-Medina, J.C., Douglas Mental Health University Institute, Department of Neurology and Neurosurgery, McGill University, 6875 LaSalle Boulevard, Montreal, QC, H4H 1R3, Canada

Morikawa, K., Department of Emergency and Critical Care Medicine, Showa University School of Medicine, 1-5-8 Hatanodai, Shinagawa-ku, Tokyo 142-8555, Japan

Murayama, T., Deparment of Pharmacology, Juntendo University School of Medicine, 2-1-1 Hongo, Bunkyo-ku, Tokyo 113-8421, Japan

Nakamachi, T., Department of Anatomy, Showa University School of Medicine, 1-5-8 Hatanotai, Shinagawa-ku, Tokyo 142-8555, Japan

Nakamura, M., Departments of Oral Anatomy and Developmental Biology, Showa University School of Dentistry, 1-5-8 Hatanodai, Shinagawa-ku, Tokyo 142-8555, Japan

Nakamura, S., Department of Oral Physiology, Showa University School of Dentistry, 1-5-8 Hatanodai, Shinagawa-ku, Tokyo 142-8555, Japan

Nakayama, K., Department of Oral Physiology, Showa University School of Dentistry, 1-5-8 Hatanodai, Shinagawa-ku, Tokyo 142-8555, Japan

Nakazato, M., Department of Division of Neurology, Respirology, Endocrinology, and Metabolism, Department of Internal Medicine, Faculty of Medicine, University of Miyazaki, 5200 Kiyotake, Miyazaki 889-1692, Japan

Norton, A.C., Department of Neurology, Beth Israel Deaconess Medical Center and Harvard Medical School, 330 Brookline Avenue, Boston, MA 02215, USA

Numazawa, S., Department of Biochemical Toxicology, School of Pharmacy, Showa University, 1-5-8 Hatanodai, Shinagawa-ku, Tokyo 142-8555, Japan

Ogawa, T., Department of Anatomy, Showa University School of Medicine, 1-5-8 Hatanodai, Shinagawa-ku, Tokyo 142-8555, Japan

Oguchi, K., Department of Pharmacology, Showa University School of Medicine, 1-5-8 Hatanodai, Shinagawa-ku, Tokyo 142-8555, Japan

Ohtaki, H., Department of Anatomy, Showa University School of Medicine, 1-5-8 Hatanodai, Shinagawa-ku, Tokyo 142-8555, Japan

Okamoto, Y., Department of Electrical, Electronics and Computer Engineering, Faculty of Engineering, Chiba Institute of Technology, 2-17-1 Tsudanuma, Narashino, Chiba 275-0016, Japan

Oyamada, H., Department of Pharmacology, Showa University School of Medicine, 1-5-8 Hatanodai, Shinagawa-ku, Tokyo 142-8555, Japan

Pan, W., Blood-Brain Barrier Group, Pennington Biomedical Research Center, Baton Rouge, LA 70808, USA

Quirion, R., Douglas Mental Health University Institute, Department of Psychiatry, McGill University, 6875 LaSalle Boulevard, Montreal, QC, H4H 1R3, Canada

Sakahara, M., Division of Molecular Biology, Department of Biochemistry and Molecular Biology, Kobe University Graduate School of Medicine, 7-5-1 Kusunoki-cho, Chuo-ku, Kobe 650-0017, Japan

Sakurai, T., Deparment of Pharmacology, Juntendo University School of Medicine, 2-1-1 Hongo, Bunkyo-ku, Tokyo 113-8421, Japan

Schlaug, G., Department of Neurology, Beth Israel Deaconess Medical Center and Harvard Medical School, 330 Brookline Avenue, Boston, MA 02215, USA

Shioda, S., Department of Anatomy, Showa University School of Medicine, 1-5-8 Hatanodai, Shinagawa-ku, Tokyo 142-8555, Japan

Shiroishi, T., Mouse Genomics Resource Laboratory, National Institute of Genetics, 1111 Yata, Mishima, Shizuoka 411-0801, Japan

Suzuki, A., Program of Gerontological Research Organization for Interdisciplinary Research, University of Tokyo, Tokyo, Japan; Beckman Institute, University of Illinois, Urbana, USA; Japan Society for the Promotion of Science

Suzuki, D., Departments of Biochemistry and Oral Anatomy and Developmental Biology, Showa University School of Dentistry, 1-5-8 Hatanodai, Shinagawa-ku, Tokyo 142-8555, Japan

Takeda, A., Department of Neurology, Showa University School of Medicine, 1-5-8 Hatanodai, Shinagawa-ku, Tokyo 142-8666, Japan

Takeda, S., Department of Orthopedic Surgery, Graduate School, Tokyo Medical and Dental University, 1-5-45 Yushima, Bunkyo-ku, Tokyo 113-8519, Japan

Takenoya, F., Department of Anatomy, Showa University School of Medicine, 1-5-8 Hatanodai, Shinagawa-ku, Tokyo 142-8555, Japan; Department of Physical Education, Hoshi University School of Pharmacy and Pharmaceutical Science, 2-4-41 Ebara, Shinagawa, Tokyo 142-8501, Japan

Taketomi, Y., Center for Biotechnology, Showa University, 1-5-8 Hatanodai, Shinagawa-ku, Tokyo 142-8555, Japan

Tamura, M., Mouse Genomics Resource Laboratory, National Institute of Genetics, 1111 Yata, Mishima, Shizuoka 411-0801, Japan

Tanaka, S., Department of Biochemical Toxicology, School of Pharmacy, Showa University, 1-5-8 Hatanodai, Shinagawa-ku, Tokyo 142-8555, Japan

Toriizuka, K., Laboratory of Pharmacognosy and Phytochemistry, School of Pharmacy, Showa University, 1-5-8 Hatanodai, Shinagawa-ku, Tokyo 142-8555, Japan

Tsumaki, N., Department of Bone and Cartilage Biology, Osaka University Graduate School of Medicine, 2-2 Yamadaoka, Suita, Osaka 565-0871, Japan

Tsuruya, N., Department of Neurology, Showa University School of Medicine, 1-5-8 Hatanodai, Shinagawa-ku, Tokyo 142-8666, Japan

Vines, B.W., Department of Neurology, Beth Israel Deaconess Medical Center and Harvard Medical School, 330 Brookline Avenue, Boston, MA 02215, USA; Institute of Mental Health, Department of Psychiatry, The University of British Columbia, 430-5950 University Boulevard, Vancouver, BC, V6T 1Z3, Canada

Yamada, A., Departments of Biochemistry, Oral Anatomy, and Developmental Biology, Showa University School of Dentistry, 1-5-8 Hatanodai, Shinagawa-ku, Tokyo 142-8555, Japan

Yamasue, H., Department of Neuropsychiatry, University of Tokyo Graduate School of Medicine, 7-3-1 Hongo, Bunkyo-ku, Tokyo 113-8655, Japan; Department of Psychiatry, Showa University School of Medicine

Yamazawa, T., Department of Molecular Cellular Pharmacology, University of Tokyo Graduate School of Medicine, 7-3-1 Hongo, Bunkyo-ku, Tokyo 113-0033, Japan

Yasuhara, R., Departments of Biochemistry, Oral Anatomy, and Developmental Biology, Showa University School of Dentistry, 1-5-8 Hatanodai, Shinagawa-ku, Tokyo 142-8555, Japan

Yofu, S., Department of Anatomy, Showa University School of Medicine, 1-5-8 Hatanodai, Shinagawa-ku, Tokyo 142-8555, Japan

Yoshida, T., Department of Biochemical Toxicology, School of Pharmacy, Showa University, 1-5-8 Hatanodai, Shinagawa-ku, Tokyo 142-8555, Japan

Color Plates

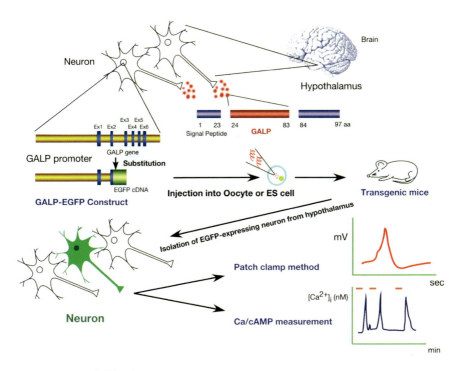

Kageyama et al. **Fig. 2.**

Strategy for analysis of GALP function.

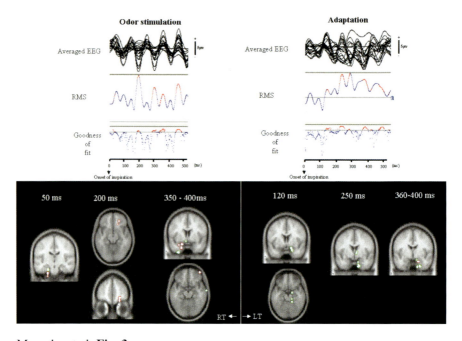

Masaoka et al. **Fig. 3**

Results of dipole analysis during odor stimulation and adaptation period.

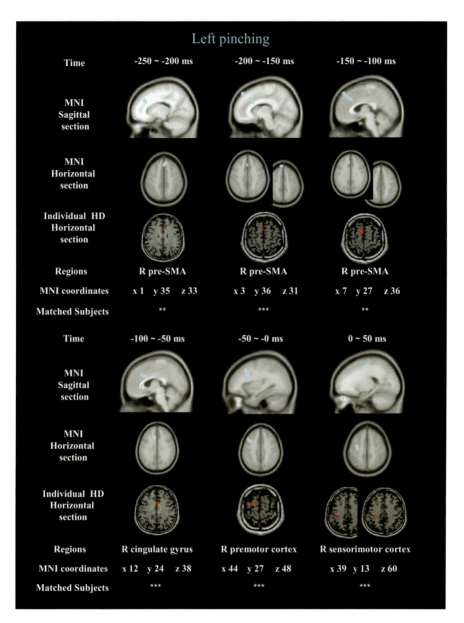

Inoue et al. **Fig. 2**

Dipole estimation of ground averaged MRCP of all the subjects incorporate with MNI standard brain by left pinching movements and typical example of dipole localization estimated from MRCP of single subject incorporate with individual head model. Regions in brain are also shown and the * stands for subjects' numbers whose dipoles appeared in each regions. Dipoles greater than 98% were indicated pre 250 to post 50 ms in order of 50 ms. Modified from Neuroscience Letter 2008, Inoue et al.

Neuropeptides and Behavior

Evolution of neuropeptide concepts illustrated by MIF-1 and MSH

Weihong Pan, Abba J. Kastin

Blood-Brain Barrier Group, Pennington Biomedical Research Center, Baton Rouge, LA 70808, USA
<e-mail> weihong.pan@pbrc.edu

Summary. Melanocyte-stimulating hormone (MSH) release-inhibiting factor (MIF)-1 is a tripeptide mainly produced by the hypothalamus. Since its discovery in 1968, MIF-1 has invoked a rich body of literature elucidating its biochemical properties, cellular actions, effects on animal behavior, and therapeutic potential in the human disorders Parkinson's disease and mental depression. The chemical synthesis of MIF-1 analogs and isolation of naturally occurring peptides with potent biological activities have yielded a family of Tyr-MIF-1 peptides. Among these, endomorphin-1 and endomorphin-2 show selective agonistic activity for the μ-opiate receptor and therapeutic potential in pain and addiction. Overall, the structural-functional analyses of MIF-1 and other members in this peptide family during the past four decades clearly demonstrate the evolution of the concepts of peptides during our lifetime. This review will summarize some of the concepts, from their initial controversy to widely accepted facts nowadays.

Keywords: peptide, concepts, MIF-1, MSH, Parkinson's disease, mental depression, antiopiate

Introduction

Melanocyte-stimulating hormone (MSH) release-inhibiting factor (MIF-1, Pro-Leu-Gly-NH$_2$,or PLG) was the first hypothalamic peptide shown to act on higher centers in the brain. It is effective in animal models of mental depression and Parkinson's disease, as well as in some patients suffering from these disorders. Many of the pharmacological studies have been reviewed recently (Pan and Kastin 2007b). In addition, a team of neurologists in Shanghai, China also performed a series of brain distribution studies of MIF-1. After intraperitoneal injection, ^{3}H-MIF-1 was rapidly distributed to rat brain, with the highest concentration in the pituitary, followed by the striatum, hypothalamus, and midbrain (Cai et al. 1989). In rats with unilateral substantia nigra lesions induced by 6-OHDA, intraperitoneal injection of MIF-1 (2 ng/kg) potentiated the effect of L-Dopa on apomorphine-induced turning. MIF-1 also reduced endorphin levels in the caudate nucleus at a dose of 20 mg/kg (Pan et al. 1985). In patients, MIF-1 reduced the side-effects and prolonged the efficacy of Madopar (levodopa + benserazide). The effect lasted 2 – 6 weeks after drug cessation (Pan 1982;Xu et al. 1986;Wang et al. 1992). The significant potentiation of the effects of Madopar by MIF-1 to reduce dyskinesia, rigidity, and tremor in these studies is consistent with what has been reported in other studies, particularly by Barbeau (1975). In his small-scale case study, "The improvement obtained in almost all (5/6) cases was of such magnitude that it far surpassed the clinical effect of any of the numerous antiparkinson drugs which we have tested in our laboratory over the past 15 years, including levodopa itself."

The isolation of MIF-1 from brain tissue was accomplished almost four decades ago. Five thousand bovine hypothalamic tissue fragments were concentrated 11,000-fold, and underwent thin layer chromatography (Schally and Kastin 1966; Nair et al. 1971). Extracts of cerebral cortex were less active than those from the hypothalamus in inhibiting MSH release. Recently, we applied a sensitive and specific triple quadrupole mass spectrometry system with QJet ion guide that clearly showed the presence of MIF-1 in the hypothalamus as well as in the striatum and elsewhere in the mouse brain (Kheterpal et al., unpublished data}. Signaling studies and biochemical analyses of synaptosomal preparations further indicated region- and cell-type specific regulation of the action of MIF-1 (Yu C, Khan R, et al., unpublished data).

1. Hypothalamic peptides can act "up" as well as "down"

The classical hypothalamic-pituitary-target organ axis involves the production of a hypothalamic releasing or inhibiting hormone, its transport to the anterior pituitary via the hypophyseal portal circulation, the release of pituitary hormone to the circulating blood where it affects its target gland, and a negative feedback on the production of pituitary and hypothalamic hormones by the target gland hormone. This pathway, although important, appears to be somewhat limited. It was shown that the same hypothalamic hormone can act on other brain regions "higher up" than the hypothalamus. This was first shown with MIF-1 (Plotnikoff et al. 1971;Kastin et al. 1978a). Many peptides can cross the blood-brain barrier (BBB) and reach brain regions other than the hypothalamus or circumventricular organs (CVOs). The anti-Parkinson's, anti-depression, and anti-opiate effects of peptides in the MIF-1 family showed that the effects of these peptides are not confined to the hypothalamus. These points will be further elaborated upon in the subsequent text.

2. Peptides in the periphery can act on the brain

It is difficult to believe that there was a time when the prevailing dogma insisted that peptides in the periphery could not have any effect whatsoever on the brain. This was not limited to those investigators who were sure that peptides couldn't cross the BBB, but extended to those who could not conceive of even indirect effects on the brain. It didn't help that some early studies using adrenocorticotropin (ACTH) or vasopressin failed to consider the secondary effects of these pituitary hormones (e.g., on adrenal steroid release and blood pressure) or the vehicle itself (Ley and Corsen 1970). The first unconfounded studies used the pituitary hormone MSH (melanocortin) to show effects on behavior and electrophysiological (EEG) responses in rats as well as human beings (Kastin et al. 1968, 1971b, 1973, 1975; Sandman et al. 1969, 1971, 1975, 1977). Many supporting studies came from the Utrecht group headed by DeWied (De Wied et al. 1974). We then dissected the effects on learning and memory to show that the process of attention was a key component (Sandman et al. 1972,1974;Miller et al. 1974). Unfortunately, Organon chose to pursue an MSH analog whose efficacy was determined by the conditioned avoidance response, rather than testing the native MSH itself which has broader effects. They failed to consider that different analogs of MSH can have differing dose-related responses in different behavioral paradigms (Miller et al. 1977;Sandman et al. 1980).

3. One peptide can exert more than one action

Two articles in *Nature* (Kastin et al. 1965, 1971a) and one in *Lancet* (Kastin et al. 1968) were the first to use the term 'extra-pigmentary' to describe the effects of MSH. Besides the behavioral and EEG effects in rats and human beings for both MSH and MIF-1, both these peptides can exert antiopiate effects, as discussed below. Moreover, luteinizing hormone-releasing hormone (LHRH) is now sometimes called gonadotropin-releasing hormone (GnRH) because of its ability to release both LH and FSH (Schally et al. 1971, 1973). Whereas MIF-1 exerts antiopiate activity, addition of a single amino acid to this tripeptide yields peptides like Tyr-MIF-1 (Tyr-Pro-Leu-Gly-amide) that can exert both opiate and antiopiate actions (Zadina et al. 1992), as does Tyr-W-MIF-1 (Tyr-Pro-Trp-Gly-amide) (Erchegyi et al. 1992;Yang and Chiu 1997). Clearly, the one hormone-one action theory died a long time ago.

4. Peptide actions can persist longer that their half-lives in blood

Although there is a general correlation of the biological action of a substance with its half life in blood, this is less applicable to peptides. Peptides in blood maintain their integrity for only a few minutes, whereas the actions mentioned above for MIF-1 and MSH can persist for several hours. This also is true for LHRH (Pfaff 1973;Moss and McCann 1973). Surprisingly, the half-life of MIF-1 in human plasma is 5 days although in rat plasma it is only a few minutes, like other small peptides including the related Tyr-MIF-1 and endomorphins (Kastin et al. 1994;Walter et al. 1975;Redding et al. 1973, 1974). Moreover, unlike many peptides, MIF-1 is active orally in rodents (Plotnikoff et al. 1973, 1974;Plotnikoff and Kastin 1974; Sharma et al. 2003) and human beings (Kastin and Barbeau 1972; Ehrensing and Kastin 1974, 1978; Barbeau et al. 1976; van der Velde 1983). Apparently the actions of a circulating peptide on the CNS are initiated very early, triggering signals that may take longer to be manifest.

5. Increased peptide doses can result in decreased effects

When we submitted our first papers showing the CNS effects of MIF-1, some referees insisted that only the linear dose-response relationship known for most substances at that time must apply to peptides. Although the mechanism for inverted-U, bell-shaped dose-response relationships remains elusive, it has become so generalized a phenomenon that Calabrese recently published 14 papers in *Crit Rev Toxicol* (volume 38, 2008) ably summarizing its occurrence in a variety of experimental and clinical situations, to which we added our commentary (Kastin and Pan 2008). He has applied the term "hormesis" to such a phenomenon. One of the examples of this phenomenon with important clinical implications is the use of MIF-1 to treat mental depression. MIF-1 exerts maximal effects in less than a week, usually 3-5 days, and these effects can persist for months, but larger doses may be less effective (Ehrensing and Kastin 1974, 1978;Ehrensing et al. 1994), as also seen in animal studies (Kastin et al. 1978b, 1984;Pan and Kastin 2007b).

6. The brain contains antiopiate peptides

Many of the concepts we have introduced into the peptide field were based on the simple idea of the efficiency of the organism. It obviously is more efficient of the body to use a peptide for more than one action than it is to create a new peptide for each desired function. This is implicit in some of the concepts discussed above. It is consistent with the multiple controlling systems involving negative and positive feedback known to occur throughout the body. Therefore, it seemed reasonable that endogenous antiopiates might exist, particularly in the brain, to modify the opiates there. The term opioid was originally introduced to indicate endogenous peptides with opiate activity, but it has been used in so many different ways that this distinction is now moot. MIF-1 was the first peptide to show antiopiate activity and introduce the concept (Kastin et al. 1979). Although it did not completely duplicate all the effects of naloxone in every situation, it functioned as an antiopiate by itself and in reversing the effects of morphine in many experimental conditions reviewed elsewhere (Pan and Kastin 2007b), as well as in a clinical study (Ehrensing et al. 1984). The concluding sentence of the abstract of the original paper predicted that antiopiate activity would be found for other endogenous peptides (Kastin et al. 1979). This prediction was later validated for peptides already known to exist, like

CCK-8, MSH, somatostatin, hemorphins, and morphiceptin, as well as for peptides such as members of the NPFF family, nociceptin/orphanin FQ, and enterostatin discovered after the antiopiate concept was established.

7. Perinatal administration of peptides exerts long-lasting effects

Most of the concepts mentioned above that we introduced into the scientific literature were met with great skepticism if not derision. Fortunately, as happens in science, they are universally appreciated now. The concept that perinatal administration of peptides can exert long-lasting effects was relatively easily accepted without much of the difficulty encountered by the other concepts. It didn't require an imaginative leap since the precedent had already been established with perinatal administration of sex steroids. It did, however, surprise some investigators who had not accepted concept number 4, above, that a peptide's half-life in blood does not necessarily correlate with its biological actions. This concept for peptides was first shown with MSH (Beckwith et al. 1977a, 1977b) and TRH (Stratton et al. 1976), and then with endorphin (Sandman et al. 1979;Moldow et al. 1981), Met-enkephalin (Kastin et al. 1980), MIF-1 (D'Amore et al. 1990), and Tyr-MIF-1 (Zadina et al. 1985, 1987), even affecting the BBB transport system for Tyr-MIF-1 (Harrison et al. 1993;Banks et al. 1996).

8. There is a specific mu-opiate receptor peptide ligand

With endogenous peptides already known to selectively bind to the delta and kappa opiate receptors in the brain, it was anticipated that there would be a peptide selectively binding to the mu site, the main receptor for the actions of morphine, since endorphin was relatively non-selective. Tyr-MIF-1, consisting of the MIF-1 tripeptide with a tyrosine at the N-terminus had some affinity for the mu-opiate site, as well as high affinity for its own site, in contrast to the lack of such binding by MIF-1. The related tetrapeptide Tyr-W-MIF-1, was isolated from bovine (Hackler et al. 1993) and human (Erchegyi et al. 1992) brain tissue and shown to be identical to Tyr-MIF-1 except for substitution of tryptophan in the third position. This tetrapeptide has about 200-fold selectivity for mu over delta and kappa opiate receptors (Zadina et al. 1994). Additional single amino acid substitutions resulted in endomorphin-1 (Tyr-Pro-Trp-Phe-amide) and, unexpectedly, endomorphin-2 (Tyr-Pro-Phe-Phe-amide), isolated from bovine

(Zadina et al. 1997) and human (Hackler et al. 1997) brain tissue with the highest affinity and selectivity for the mu opiate receptor. About 500 papers with the endomorphins have substantiated their role.

9. A peptide's name does not restrict its actions

Perhaps some of the reason why these concepts were not introduced earlier may involve the bias toward thinking of the functions of a peptide by the action by which it was first described. For example, MSH obviously does more than stimulate melanocytes, especially in mammals, LHRH releases FSH as well as LH, orexin affects sleep and food ingestion, and somatostatin inhibits more peptides than just growth hormone (somatotropin). It is unfortunate that some young investigators seem to be so intimidated by the name of the peptide that they are not inclined to think "out of the box" concerning its other possible roles.

10. Peptides can cross the blood-brain barrier

This concept is listed last because it is a subject of continuing interest to so many investigators since we introduced the concept about three decades ago. Initially controversial, like so many of the concepts listed above, it succeeded relatively rapidly to overcome the existing dogma. Skepticism about the ability of peptides to cross the BBB was related in part to the concept (number 4) discussed above. Even the "blue-ribbon" advisory panel to NIH stated, "Since the half-life of (peptides) is short, it is unlikely that significant entry occurs into brain" (1981). MIF-1 is rapidly transported into brain from blood by a partially saturable system whereas Tyr-MIF-1 only enters slowly by passive diffusion. By contrast, Tyr-MIF-1 has a saturable transport system out of the brain that is not shared by MIF-1 but is shared by Met-enkephalin (Banks and Kastin 1984;Banks et al. 1986,1987).

The proton-dependent peptide transporters PEPT1 and PEPT2 mediate cellular uptake of di- and tripeptides as well as a variety of drug molecules. It is known that PEPT2 is present and functional at the blood-cerebrospinal fluid barrier. The transport kinetics of a model dipeptide glycylsarcosine (GlySar) in primary culture of choroid plexus epithelial cells show inhibition by di/tripeptides, carnosine and alpha-amino cephalosporins, but are unaffected by amino acids, cephalosporins lacking an alpha-amino group, and organic anions and cations (Shu et al. 2002). It is not clear whether the

MIF-1 peptides use PEPT2. Nonetheless, it seems that P-glycoproteins (P-gp) play no role in the efflux transport of Tyr-MIF-1 or the endomorphins, shown by use of knockout mice deficient in P-gp or in the presence of cyclosporin A, an inhibitor of the P-gp system (Kastin et al. 2002;Somogyvari-Vigh et al. 2004).

The pharmacokinetic studies of the MIF-1 family of peptides crossing the BBB illustrate that a peptide may permeate the BBB to exert potent biological actions. Following this, there have been a series of studies with bioactive peptides (Pan and Kastin 2004b, 2007a;Yu et al. 2004;Pan et al. 2005; 2006b). Besides pharmacokinetic analyses of the permeability, there are mechanistic studies on the intracellular trafficking and transcytosis. The peptide studies also led to characterization of the permeation of larger proteins, especially the polypeptide neurotrophins and cytokines (Pan et al. 1998, 2006a;Pan and Kastin 2004b).

The BBB interfaces the parenchyma of brain and spinal cord and its supplying capillary vessels. The structural components are microvessel endothelial cells, pericytes, astrocytic endfeet, and extracellular matrix. The endothelial cells are joined by tight junctions, lined by a continuous basement membrane, and have reduced pinocytic vesicles and increased metabolic and enzymatic activity. These structural features are involved in the relative impermeability of the BBB to large proteins in the circulating blood. However, there are many instances in which peptides and proteins produced in the periphery have CNS effects, and most of such actions are mediated by the BBB. Many peptides cross the BBB by passive diffusion, based on physicochemical properties such as lipophilicity, hydrogen bonding, and conformation. However, some peptides cross the BBB by saturable transport systems that may or may not involve receptor mediated transport. Moreover, some efflux systems from brain to blood are also saturable. There are two principal ways by which cytokines interact with the BBB: (a) their transport or transcytosis across the endothelial cells that are the structural backbone of the BBB (Banks et al. 1991; Gutierrez et al. 1993; Pan and Kastin 2004a; Pan et al. 2007a; Yu et al. 2007b) and (b) their actions on these endothelial cells which result in altered endothelial function, cytotoxicity, or cell proliferation (Yu et al. 2007a, 2007c, 2007d).

Besides the BBB, peptides, polypeptides, and proteins are also known to interact with the blood-cerebrospinal fluid barrier and the circumventricular organs. Nonetheless, in the case of MIF-1, there appears to be more CNS activation shown by c-Fos immunoreactivity in mouse brain after intravenous delivery of MIF-1 than after intracerebroventricular delivery (Yu C et al., unpublished data).

Recent progress with understanding of the BBB has involved interactions between MSH and leptin within the BBB endothelial cells. Cerebral endothelial cells, the main constituent of the BBB, show co-expression of the receptors for leptin and melanocortin, suggesting possible interactions between leptin and MSH signaling. In cellular models in which mouse ObRb, MC3R or MC4R were expressed at high levels after transient transfection, we measured leptin-induced activation of signal transducers and activators of transcription (STAT)-3. Reciprocally, we also measured αMSH-induced production of cAMP. For central effects of feeding, ObRb, not a G-protein coupled receptor, is the main signaling receptor for leptin while MC3R and MC4R, G-protein coupled receptors, are the main receptors for αMSH. In the endothelial cell model, αMSH potentiated the STAT3 activation induced by leptin, while leptin had only a minor effect in increasing αMSH-initiated cAMP production downstream to MC3R. The interaction between leptin and melanocortin receptors is similar to that shown between ObRb and corticotropin-releasing hormone receptors for urocortin (Pan et al. 2007c). This suggests a possible generalized cooperation of ObRb and G-protein coupled receptors (Zhang Y et al., unpublished data). Such novel potentiation in cellular signaling may have considerable biological implications.

11. Philosophical musings

All these concepts are clear now, but some lessons can be gleaned from them. As Richard Conniff stated in the June 2008 issue of the *Smithsonian*, "Ideas that seem obvious in retrospect are anything but, in real life". An adaptation of Schopenhauer's evaluation of discovery has it going through three stages of being ridiculed, opposed, and finally accepted as self-evident. Considering how difficult it was for some of these concepts to gain acceptance, investigators, especially young ones, might benefit from heeding the recommendation attributed to Alexander Fleming: "Don't let your mind be cluttered up with prevailing doctrine". Similarly, Kiekegaard gave this admonition: "There are two ways to be fooled: one is to believe what isn't so; the other is to refuse to believe what is so."

Acknowledgement
Current grant support to the authors is provided by NIH (DK54880, NS45751, NS46528, and NS62291). We thank our former laboratory members and collaborators for much of the work discussed here, particularly Drs. Curt A. Sandman, Richard and Gayle Olson, James E. Zadina and William A. Banks. We also thank Drs. Seiji Shioda and Rudolph H. Ehrensing for inspiring this longitudinal review of MIF-1 and MSH.

References

An Evaluation of Research Needs in Endocrinology and Metabolic Diseases. Vol IV, 495. 1981. Advisory Report to the NIH

Banks WA, Kastin AJ (1984) A brain-to-blood carrier-mediated transport system for small, N-tyrosinated peptides. Pharmacol Biochem Behav 21:943-946

Banks WA, Kastin AJ, Fischman AJ, Coy DH, Strauss SL (1986) Carrier-mediated transport of enkephalins and N-Tyr-MIF-1 across blood-brain barrier. Am J Physiol 251:E477-E482

Banks WA, Kastin AJ, Michals EA (1987) Tyr-MIF-1 and Met-enkephalin share a saturable blood-brain barrier transport system. Peptides 8:899-903

Banks WA, Kastin AJ, Harrison LM, Zadina JE (1996) Perinatal treatment of rats with opiates affects the development of the blood-brain barrier transport system PTS-1. Neurotoxicol Teratol 18:711-715

Banks WA, Ortiz L, Plotkin SR, Kastin AJ (1991) Human interleukin (IL) 1a, murine IL-1α and murine IL-1β are transported from blood to brain in the mouse by a shared saturable mechanism. J Pharmacol Exp Ther 259:988-996

Barbeau A (1975) Potentiation of levodopa effect by intravenous L-prolyl-L-leucyl-glycine amide in man. Lancet 2:683-684

Barbeau A, Roy M, Kastin AJ (1976) Double-blind evaluation of oral L-prolyl-L-leucyl-glycine amide in Parkinson's disease. Can Med Assoc J 114:120-122

Beckwith BW, O'Quin RK, Petro MS, Kastin AJ, Sandman CA (1977a) The effects of neonatal injections of α-MSH on the open field behavior of juvenile and adult rats. Physiol Psychol 5:295-299

Beckwith BW, Sandman CA, Hothersall D, Kastin AJ (1977b) Influence of neonatal injections of α-MSH on learning, memory and attention in rats. Physiol Behav 18:63-71

Cai H, Xu D, Yu H, Wang Z (1989) The distribution of PLG in rat brain. Chinese J Neurol Psychiat 5:292-293

D'Amore A, Pieretti S, Palazzesi S, Pezzini G, Chiarotti F, Scorza T, Loizzo A (1990) MIF-1 can accelerate neuromotor, EEG and behavioral development in mice. Peptides 11:527-532

De Wied D, Bohus B, Wimersma Greidanus TB (1974) The hypothalamo-neurohypophyseal system and the preservation of conditioned avoidance behavior in rats. Prog Brain Res 41:417-428

Ehrensing RH, Kastin AJ (1974) Melanocyte-stimulating hormone-release inhibiting hormone as an anti-depressant: a pilot study. Arch Gen Psychiat 30:63-65

Ehrensing RH, Kastin AJ (1978) Dose-related biphasic effect of prolyl-leucyl-glycinamide (MIF-I) in depression. Am J Psychiatry 135:562-566

Ehrensing RH, Kastin AJ, Michell GF (1984) Antagonism of morphine analgesia by prolyl-leucyl-glycinamide (MIF-1) in humans. Pharmacol Biochem Behav 21:975-978

Ehrensing RH, Kastin AJ, Wurzlow GF, Michell GF, Mebane AH (1994) Improvement in major depression after low subcutaneous doses of MIF-1. J Affect Disord 31:227-233

Erchegyi J, Kastin AJ, Zadina JE (1992) Isolation of a novel tetrapeptide with opiate and antiopiate activity from human brain cortex: Tyr-Pro-Trp-Gly-NH$_2$ (Tyr-W-MIF-1). Peptides 13:623-632

Gutierrez EG, Banks WA, Kastin AJ (1993) Murine tumor necrosis factor alpha is transported from blood to brain in the mouse. J Neuroimmunol 47:169-176

Hackler L, Kastin AJ, Erchegyi J, Zadina JE (1993) Isolation of Tyr-W-MIF-1 from bovine hypothalami. Neuropeptides 24:159-164

Hackler L, Zadina JE, Ge L-J, Kastin AJ (1997) Isolation of relatively large amounts of endomorphin-1 and endomorphin-2 from human brain cortex. Peptides 18:1635-1639

Harrison LM, Zadina JE, Banks WA, Kastin AJ (1993) Effects of neonatal treatment with Tyr-MIF-1, morphiceptin and morphine on development, tail flick, and blood-brain barrier transport. Dev Brain Res 75:207-212

Kastin AJ, Abel DA, Ehrensing RH, Coy DH, Graf MV (1984) Tyr-MIF-1 and MIF-1 are active in the water wheel test for antidepressant drugs. Pharmacol Biochem Behav 21:767-771

Kastin AJ, Arimura A, Schally AV, Miller M (1971a) Mass-action type, direct feedback control of pituitary MSH release. Nature 231:29-30

Kastin AJ, Barbeau A (1972) Preliminary clinical studies with L-prolyl-L-leucyl-glycine amide in Parkinson's disease. Can Med Assoc J 107:1079-1081

Kastin AJ, Coy DH, Schally AV, Miller LH (1978a) Peripheral administration of hypothalamic peptides results in CNS changes. Pharmacol Res Commun 10:293-312

Kastin AJ, Fasold MB, Zadina JE (2002) Endomorphins, Met-Enkephalin, Tyr-MIF-1, and the P-glycoprotein efflux system. Drug Metab Disp 30:231-234

Kastin AJ, Hahn K, Erchegyi J, Zadina JE, Hackler L, Palmgren M, Banks WA (1994) Differential metabolism of Tyr-MIF-1 and MIF-1 in rat and human plasma. Biochem Pharmacol 47:699-709

Kastin AJ, Kostrzewa RM, Schally AV, Coy DH (1980) Neonatal administration of Met-enkephalin facilitates maze performance of adult rats. Pharmacol Biochem Behav 13:883-886

Kastin AJ, Kullander S, Borglin N, Dyster-Aas K, Dahlberg B, Ingvar D, Krakau C, Miller M, Bowers C, Schally AV (1968) Extrapigmentary effects of MSH in amenorrheic women. Lancet 1:1007-1010

Kastin AJ, Miller LH, Gonzalez-Barcena D, Hawley WD, Dyster-Aas K, Schally AV, Velasco-Parra ML, Velasco M (1971b) Psycho-physiologic correlates of MSH activity in man. Physiol Behav 7:893-896

Kastin AJ, Miller LH, Nockton R, Sandman CA, Schally AV, Stratton LO (1973) Behavioral aspects of MSH. Prog Brain Res 39:461-470

Kastin AJ, Olson RD, Ehrensing RH, Berzas MC, Schally AV, Coy DH (1979) MIF-1's differential actions as an opiate antagonist. Pharmacol Biochem Behav 11:721-723

Kastin AJ, Pan W (2008) Peptides and hormesis. Crit Rev Toxicol 38:629-631

Kastin AJ, Sandman CA, Stratton LO, Schally AV, Miller LH (1975) Behavioral and electrographic changes in rat and man after MSH. Prog Brain Res 42:143-150

Kastin AJ, Scollan EL, Ehrensing RH, Schally AV, Coy DH (1978b) Enkephalin and other peptides reduce passiveness. Pharmacol Biochem Behav 9:515-519

Kastin AJ, Schally AV, Yajima H, Kubo K (1965) Melanocyte stimulating hormone activity of synthetic MSH and ACTH peptides in vivo and in vitro. Nature 207:978-979

Ley F, Corsen J (1970) Effects of ACTH and zinc phosphate vehicle on shuttlebox CAR. Psychon Sci 20:307-309

Miller LH, Kastin AJ, Sandman CA, Fink M, Van Veen WJ (1974) Polypeptide influence on attention, memory, and anxiety in man. Pharmacol Biochem Behav 2:663-668

Miller L, Fischer S, Groves G, Rudrauff M, Kastin AJ (1977) MSH/ACTH 4-10 influences on the CAR in human subjects: a negative finding. Pharmacol Biochem Behav 7:417-419

Moldow RL, Kastin AJ, Hollander C, Coy DH, Sandman CA (1981) Brain ß-endorphin-like immunoreactivity in adult rats given ß-endorphin neonatally. Brain Res Bull 7:683-686

Moss RL, McCann SM (1973) Induction of mating behavior in rats by luteinizing hormone-releasing factor. Science 181:177

Nair RMG, Kastin AJ, Schally AV (1971) Isolation and structure of hypothalamic MSH release-inhibiting hormone. Biochem Biophys Res Commun 43:1376-1425

Pan J (1982) Effect of PLG on Parkinson's disease. J Internatl Neurol Neurosurg 5:2

Pan J, Xu D, Zhao Y, Yu H (1985) Mechanisms of the anti-Parkinson's effect of PLG. Chinese J Neurol Psychiat 18:205-208

Pan W, Kastin AJ (2004a) Transport of cytokines and neurotrophins across the blood-brain barrier and their regulation after spinal cord injury. In: Sharma HS, Westman J (eds) Blood-Spinal Cord and Brain Barriers in Health and Disease. Elsevier, San Diego, CA, pp. 395-407

Pan W, Kastin AJ (2004b) Why study transport of peptides and proteins at the neurovascular interface. Brain Res Rev 46:32-43

Pan W, Kastin AJ (2007a) Adipokines and the blood-brain barrier. Peptides 28:1317-1330

Pan W, Kastin AJ, Daniel J, Yu C, Basbaum A, Baryshnikova LM, von Bartheld CS (2007a) TNF alpha trafficking in cerebral vascular endothelial cells. J Neuroimmunol 185:47-56

Pan W, Xiang S, Tu H, Kastin AJ (2006a) Cytokines interact with the blood-brain barrier. In: Dermietzel R, Spray DC, Nedergaard M (eds) Blood-Brain Barrier Interfaces: From Ontogeny to Artificial Barriers. Wiley- VCH, Weinheim, Germany, pp. 247-264

Pan W, Yu Y, Cain CM, Nyberg F, Couraud P, Kastin AJ (2005) Permeation of growth hormone across the blood-brain barrier. Endocrinology 146:4898-4904

Pan W, Yu Y, Nyberg F, Kastin AJ (2006b) Growth hormone, insulin, and insulin-like growth factor-1: Do they interact at the blood-brain barrier? In: Nyberg F (ed) The Somatotropic Axis in Brain Function. Elsevier, San Diego, CA, pp. 75-79

Pan W, Banks WA, Kastin AJ (1998) Permeability of the blood-brain/spinal cord barrier to neurotrophins. Brain Res 788:87-94

Pan W, Kastin AJ (2007b) From MIF-1 to endomorphin: the Tyr-MIF-1 family of peptides. Peptides 28:2411-2434

Pan W, Tu H, Hsuchou H, Daniel J, Kastin AJ (2007c) Unexpected amplification of leptin-induced Stat3 signaling by urocortin: implications for obesity. J Mol Neurosci 33:232-238

Pfaff DW (1973) Luteinizing hormone-releasing factor potentiates lordosis behavior in hypophysectomized ovariectomized female rats. Science 182:1148-1149

Plotnikoff NP, Kastin AJ (1974) Oxotremorine antagonism by prolyl-leucyl-glycine amide administered by different routes and with several anticholinergics. Pharmacol Biochem Behav 2:417-419

Plotnikoff NP, Kastin AJ, Anderson MS, Schally AV (1971) DOPA potentiation by a hypothalamic factor, α-MSH release-inhibiting hormone (MIF). Life Sci 10:1279-1283

Plotnikoff NP, Kastin AJ, Anderson MS, Schally AV (1973) Deserpidine antagonism by a tripeptide, L-prolyl-L-leucylglycinamide. Neuorendocrinology 11:67-71

Plotnikoff NP, Minard FN, Kastin AJ (1974) DOPA potentiation in ablated animals and brain levels of biogenic amines in intact animals after prolyl-leucylglycinamide. Neuroendocrinology 14:271-279

Redding TW, Kastin AJ, Gonzalez-Barcena D, Coy DH, Hirotsu Y, Ruelas J, Schally AV (1974) The disappearance, excretion, and metabolism of tritiated prolyl-leucyl-glycinamide in man. Neuroendocrinology 16:119-126

Redding TW, Kastin AJ, Nair RMG, Schally AV (1973) The distribution, half-life, and excretion of ^{14}C and ^{3}H-labeled L-prolyl-L-leucyl-glycinamide in the rat. Neuroendocrinology 11:92-100

Sandman CA, Beckwith BE, Kastin AJ (1980) Are learning and attention related to the sequence of amino acids in ACTH/MSH peptides? Peptides 1:277-280

Sandman CA, Beckwith W, Gittis M, Kastin AJ (1974) Melanocyte-stimulating hormone (MSH) and overtraining effects on extradimensional shift (EDS) learning. Physiol Behav 13:163-166

Sandman CA, Denman PM, Miller LH, Knott JR, Schally AV, Kastin AJ (1971) Electroencephalographic measures of melanocyte stimulating hormone activity. J Comp Physiol Psychol 76:103-109

Sandman CA, George J, McCanne TR, Nolan JD, Kaswan J, Kastin AJ (1977) MSH/ACTH 4-10 influences behavioral and physiological measures of attention. J Clin Endocrinol Metab 44:884-891

Sandman CA, George JM, Nolan JD, Van Riezen H, Kastin AJ (1975) Enhancement of attention in man with ACTH/MSH 4-10. Physiol Behav 15:427-431

Sandman CA, Kastin AJ, Schally AV (1969) Melanocyte-stimulating hormone and learned appetitive behavior. Experientia 25:1001-1002

Sandman CA, McGivern RF, Berka C, Walker M, Coy DH, Kastin AJ (1979) Neonatal administration of β-endorphin produces "chronic" insensitivity to thermal stimuli. Life Sci 25:1755-1760

Sandman CA, Miller LH, Kastin AJ, Schally AV (1972) A neuroendocrine influence on attention and memory. J Comp Physiol Psychol 80:54-58

Schally AV, Arimura A, Kastin AJ (1973) Hypothalamic regulating hormones. Science 179:341-350

Schally AV, Arimura A, Kastin AJ, Matsuo H, Baba Y, Redding TW, Nair RMG, Debeljuk L, White W (1971) Gonadotropin-releasing hormone: one polypeptide regulates the secretion of LH and FSH. Science 173:1036- 1038

Schally AV, Kastin AJ (1966) Purification of a bovine hypothalamic factor which elevates pituitary MSH levels in rats. Endocrinology 79:768-772

Sharma S, Paladino P, Gabriele J, Saeedi H, Henry P, Chang M, Mishra RK, Johnson RL (2003) Pro-Leu-glycinamide and its peptidomimetic, PAOPA, attenuate haloperidol induced vacuous chewing movements in rat: A model of human tardive dyskinesia. Peptides 24:313-319

Shu C, Shen H, Teuscher NS, Lorenzi PJ, Keep RF, Smith DE (2002) Role of PEPT2 in peptide/mimetic trafficking at the blood-cerebrospinal fluid barrier: studies in rat choroid plexus epithelial cells in primary culture. J Pharmacol Exp Ther 301:820-829

Somogyvari-Vigh A, Kastin AJ, Liao J, Zadina JE, Pan W (2004) Endomorphins exit the brain by a saturable efflux system at the basolateral surface of cerebral endothelial cells. Exp Brain Res 156:224-230

Stratton LO, Gibson CA, Kolar KG, Kastin AJ (1976) Neonatal treatment with TRH affects development, learning, and emotionality in the rat. Pharmacol Biochem Behav 5(Suppl. 1):65-67

van der Velde CD (1983) Rapid clinical effectiveness of MIF-I in the treatment of major depressive illness. Peptides 4:297-300

Walter R, Neidle A, Marks N (1975) Significant differences in the degradation of Pro-Leu-Gly-NH$_2$ by human serum and that of other species. Proc Soc Exp Biol Med 148:98-103

Wang Z, Xu D, Yu H, Chen S, Tang G, Pan J (1992) Therapeutic effects of PLG in Parkinson's disease. Shanghai Med J 3:15

Xu D, Yu H, Chen S, Pan J (1986) Preliminary report on the effect of PLG (MIF-1) in the treatment of Parkinson's disease. Acta Universitatis Medicinalis Secondae Shanghai 4:328-331

Yang Y, Chiu T (1997) Opioid and antiopioid actions of Tyr-MIF-1, Tyr-W-MIF-1 and hemorphin-4 on rat locus coeruleus neurons: intracellular recording in vitro. Chin J Physiol 40:131-135

Yu C, Pan W, Tu H, Waters S, Kastin AJ (2007a) TNF activates p-glycoprotein in cerebral microvascular endothelial cells. Cell Physiol Biochem 20:853-858

Yu C, Kastin AJ, Ding Y, Pan W (2007b) Gamma glutamyl transpeptidase is a dynamic indicator of endothelial response to stroke. Exp Neurol 203:116-122

Yu C, Kastin AJ, Pan W (2007c) TNF reduces LIF endocytosis despite increasing NFkappaB-mediated gp130 expression. J Cell Physiol 213:161-166

Yu C, Kastin AJ, Tu H, Pan W (2007d) Opposing effects of proteasomes and lysosomes on LIFR: modulation by TNF. J Mol Neurosci 32:80-89

Yu Y, Jawa A, Pan W, Kastin AJ (2004) Effects of peptides, with emphasis on feeding, pain, and behavior: A 5-year (1999-2003) review of publications in Peptides. Peptides 25:2257-2289

Zadina JE, Hackler L, Ge L-J, Kastin AJ (1997) A potent and selective endogenous agonist for the mu-opiate receptor. Nature 386:499-502

Zadina JE, Kastin AJ, Coy DH, Adinoff BA (1985) Developmental, behavioral, and opiate receptor changes after prenatal or postnatal β-endorphin, CRF, or Tyr-MIF-1. Psychoneuroendocrinology 10:367-383

Zadina JE, Kastin AJ, Ge L-J, Hackler L (1994) *Mu*, *delta*, and *kappa* opiate receptor binding of Tyr-MIF-1 and of Tyr-W-MIF-1, its active fragments, and two potent analogs. Life Sci 55:PL461-PL466

Zadina JE, Kastin AJ, Kersh D, Wyatt A (1992) Tyr-MIF-1 and hemorphin can act as opiate agonists as well as antagonists in the guinea pig ileum. Life Sci 51:869-885

Zadina JE, Kastin AJ, Manasco PK, Pignatiello MF, Nastiuk KL (1987) Long-term hyperalgesia by neonatal β-endorphin and morphiceptin is blocked by neonatal Tyr-MIF-1. Brain Res 409:10-18

Increased leptin supply to hypothalamus by gene therapy confers life-long benefits on energy homeostasis, disease cluster of metabolic syndrome- diabetes type 1 and 2, dyslipidemia and cardiovascular ailments- and bone remodeling

Satya P. Kalra, Ph.D.

Distinguished Professor, Department of Neuroscience, University of Florida College of Medicine, McKnight Brain Institute, P.O. Box 100244, Gainesville, FL, 32610-0244, United States
Email: skalra@mbi.ufl.edu, Fax: 352 294-0191

Summary. Leptin insufficiency in the hypothalamus is causally linked to increased fat accrual, diseases of the metabolic syndrome, skeletal abnormalities and shortened life-span. We show that leptin sufficiency attained with hypothalamic leptin gene therapy (i) suppressed food intake, the age-related and energy enriched diet-induced fat accrual, and dyslipidemia, (ii) attenuated episodic insulin secretion and enhanced insulin sensitivity, (iii) enhanced glucose tolerance and maintained euglycemia by concurrently stimulating glucose metabolism and non-shivering thermogenesis, even in the absence of circulating insulin, and (iv) augmented ghrelin secretion. Aside from these metabolic benefits, similar optimal leptin sufficiency in the hypothalamus (i) decreased risks for cardiovascular diseases as indicated by suppression of circulating levels of the systemic pro-inflammatory markers, C-reactive protein and interleukin-6, and hyperglycemia-induced risk factors for cardiomyopathy, (ii) improved bone health by promoting growth of long bones and reduction of cancellous bone volume in association with increased release of osteoblast-specific osteocalcin, and (iii) reduced early mortality and doubled the life-span of obese *ob/ob* mice. On the basis of these global long-lasting health benefits, we advocate clinical testing of central leptin gene therapy or of long acting leptin mimetics to prevent life-threatening pathophysiologic sequalae attending the worldwide epidemic of obesity and the metabolic syndrome.

Key words. Gene therapy, Hypothalamus, Obesity, Metabolic syndrome, Skeleton, Life-span

1 Historical

The potent appetite stimulating effects of hypothalamic neuropeptide Y (NPY) were discovered in the mid 1980s (Clark et al. 1984). Subsequently, a concerted effort led to deciphering of a distinct circuitry in the hypothalamus that regulates energy intake and expenditure on a moment-to-moment basis (Kalra et al. 1999, 2003). This interconnected network, primarily driven by the NPY expressing pathway, is composed of orexigenic and anorexigenic peptidergic circuitries that span the arcuate nucleus (ARC), medial preoptic area (MPOA), paraventricular nucleus (PVN), ventromedial hypothalamus (VMH) and lateral hypothalamus (LH) in the diencephalon (Kalra et al. 1999, 2003). Disruption in signaling in any component of this NPY regulatory network invariably leads to unremitting hyperphagia, abnormal rate of fat accumulation and the attendant disease cluster of metabolic syndrome and shortened life-span (Dube et al. 2007; Kalra 2008b; Kalra et al. 2003).

A further insight into the working of the NPY circuitry in maintaining energy homeostasis was gained after isolation and characterization of the anorexigenic hormone leptin produced by adipocytes, and the orexigenic hormone ghrelin produced by the stomach (Friedman and Halaas 1998; Kalra et al. 2003; Otukonyong et al. 2005b). That a dynamic minute-to-minute interplay of these two afferent signals to the hypothalamic NPY network sustain energy homeostasis was then uncovered (Kalra 2008b; Kalra et al. 2003, 2009; Otukonyong et al. 2005a; Ueno et al. 2004). The current view holds that leptin is a primary peripheral signal that imposes a stable tonic restraint on hypothalamic circuitry by a three prong control: one, by regulating the release and action of orexigenic and anorexigenic hypothalamic peptides, two, by directly countering the appetite stimulating action of ghrelin in the hypothalamus and, three, by restraining ghrelin synthesis and release into the peripheral circulation from oxyntic glands of the stomach (Kalra 2008b; Kalra et al. 2003, 2005; Ueno et al. 2004).

Finally, deeper understanding of the hypothalamic control of energy homeostasis was sparked by comprehensive new information on dynamic changes in leptin transport to hypothalamic targets across the blood brain barrier (BBB) enforced on a daily basis by aging, metabolic and nutritional imbalance (Banks et al. 1999; Kalra 2008a; Kastin and Pan 2006).

This fundamental new knowledge of the brain-body dialogue coupled with global health benefits observed after application of leptin gene therapy in the hypothalamus (Kalra and Kalra 2005), was recently synthesized into a "Central Leptin Insufficiency Syndrome" formulation to explain the underlying causality of the worldwide pandemic of obesity and attendant disease cluster of metabolic syndrome, and early mortality (Fig. 1, Boghossian et al. 2007; Kalra 2008a; Olshansky et al. 2005).

Consequently, this article presents a brief collation of results obtained after application of hypothalamic leptin gene therapy in wild type (WT), obese young and aging rodents, and transgenic mice afflicted with excess fat accretion, dyslipidemia, type 1 and 2 diabetes, cardiovascular diseases and bone growth abnormalities and, thereby, faced with the impending shortened life-span.

2 Obesity Burden

Epidemiological reports have amply affirmed that a major contemporary challenge for the scientific and medical communities worldwide is to drastically curb the accelerating rate of obesity and to curtail the escalating medical costs of treating obesity-dependent diseases. A disease cluster of the metabolic syndrome, notably, dyslipidemia, type 2 diabetes, hypertension, kidney and liver dysfunction on one hand, and neural diseases, drug addiction, Alzheimer's disease, infertility, sleep apnea, some cancers, and early mortality on the other, encompass the obesity burden (Boghossian et al. 2007; Briley and Szczech 2006; Brownlee 2005; Correia and Rahmouni 2006; Kalra 2008a; Olshansky et al. 2005). Changes in lifestyle, voluntary caloric restriction and diverse ways to expend energy at accelerated rate on a daily basis, are the current interventional therapies advocated to forestall the rapid diet-induced and progressive age-related obesity (Kalra 2008a,b; Kalra and Kalra 2005; Olshansky et al. 2005). Pharmacological approaches available to reliably curb obesity on a long-term basis are extremely limited (Kalra and Kalra 2005; Olshansky et al. 2005). An evaluation of the impact on energy balance and multiple risk factors of obesity after modification of the crosstalk between fat and hypothalamus with the aid of leptin gene therapy, has identified a novel therapeutic modality capable of remedying the environmentally-induced imbalance in energy intake and expenditure and, thereby, successfully impede the obesity scourge (Kalra 2008a,b; Kalra and Kalra 2005).

3 Impact of Central Leptin Gene Therapy

We have employed gene transfer technology to introduce leptin gene in hypothalamic targets in attempts to circumvent hypothalamic leptin insufficiency that develops either gradually or rapidly due to aging, life-style and nutritional modifications (Dhillon et al. 2000, 2001; Kalra and Kalra 2005). Since recombinant adeno-associated virus (rAAV), a nonpathogenic and non-immunogenic vector, has multiple advantages over other viral vectors, including its ability to transduce expression selectively in neurons for the lifetime of cells, this vector was engineered to encode leptin gene (rAAV-lep, Dhillon et al. 2000, 2001; Kalra and Kalra 2005). Although systemic injection of rAAV-lep was found to be effective in reinstating homeostasis in leptin mutant *ob/ob* mice, this procedure was considered unsuitable because of the attending hyperleptinemia, the pleiotropic nature of leptin, and development of imperviousness of BBB to leptin in response to hyperleptinemia (Banks et al. 1999; Dhillon et al. 2000, 2001; Kalra and Kalra 2005; Kastin and Pan 2006). Therefore, we undertook to enhance leptin expression selectively in the hypothalamus after a single intracerebroventricular (icv) injection or microinjection into discrete hypothalamic sites of rAAV-lep (Bagnasco et al. 2002; Beretta et al 2002; Dhillon et al. 2000, 2001). The outcome of these series of experiments conducted in our laboratory are presented below.

3.1 Energy Homeostasis

A single icv injection of rAAV-lep to stably deliver biologically active leptin selectively at leptin-target sites in prepubertal and adult WT rodents, consuming either normal rodent chow diet or calorie-enriched diet, rapidly decreased food intake (FI) and contemporaneously, augmented non-shivering thermogenic energy expenditure for the duration of the experiment, lasting from weeks to lifetime. This combined impact on energy intake and expenditure of central leptin gene therapy prevented the age-related and energy-enriched diet-induced obesity and maintained reduced body weight (BW) for the entire duration of the experiment (Bagnasco et al. 2002; Beretta et al. 2002; Boghossian et al. 2007; Dhillon et al. 2001; Kalra and Kalra 2005). Indeed, the efficacy of the central leptin gene therapy on weight homeostasis persisted through various phases of reproduction, lactation and post-lactation and, intriguingly, it was apparent in the F1 generation (Lecklin et al. 2005). Additionally, existence of those leptin hypothalamic neuronal targets that specifically regulate energy expenditure were found in the MPOA, and were distinct from those involved in control of energy intake located caudally in the ARC-PVN axis, VMH and LH (Bagnasco et al. 2002).

3.2 Adiposity, Hormonal and Metabolic Variables

Sustenance of reduced BW in rAAV-lep treated rodents was found to be primarily due to reduced rate of fat deposition, a response that also contributed to decreases in circulating adipokines, adiponectin, tumor necrosis factor-β, cholesterol, free fatty acids and triglycerides (Bagnasco et al. 2002; Beretta et al. 2002; Boghossian et al. 2006, 2007; Dhillon et al. 2001; Kalra 2008a; Kalra and Kalra 2005). In marked contrast, icv rAAV-lep injection reliably augmented gastric ghrelin secretion, a stimulatory response attributable to diminution in leptin restraint on ghrelin secretion at the level of gastric oxyntic glands, and blockade by leptin of ghrelin-induced appetite through a hypothalamic action (Bagnasco et al. 2002; Kalra 2008b; Kalra et al. 2003; Lecklin et al. 2005; Ueno et al. 2004). It is highly likely that this increased ghrelin secretion may play a prominent role in life-span extension by rAAV-lep (Boghossian et al. 2007; Rigamonti et al. 2002).

4 Diabetes type 1 and type 2

Since etiological sequalae that underlie the pathophysiology of type 1 and type 2 diabetes are distinct, the therapeutic modalities available to ameliorate hyperglycemia for these two diseases are distinct and diverse (Boghossian et al. 2006; Kalra 2008a,b; Kalra and Kalra 2005; Ueno et al. 2006) . Our investigation of the dynamic working of the pancreatic insulin-glucose axis in response to hypothalamic leptin gene therapy has, quite unexpectedly, uncovered the therapeutic ability of stable optimal leptin supply to impel euglycemia in rodents afflicted with either type 1 or type 2 diabetes (Bagnasco et al. 2002; Boghossian et al. 2006, 2007; Kalra 2008a). The efficacy of central leptin gene therapy was tested in two non-obese models of type 1 diabetes (Boghossian et al. 2007; Hidaka et al. 2002; Kalra 2008b; Kojima et al, 2009; Ueno et al. 2006; Yoshioka et al. 1997). A single icv injection of rAAV-lep maintained euglycemia in hyperglycemic diabetic mice with insulitis induced by streptozotocin (Hidaka et al. 2002; Kojima et al. 2009). Furthermore, sustenance of euglycemia by one rAAV-lep injection completely blocked the early mortality seen normally in streptozotocin-pretreated mice (Hidaka et al. 2002; Kojima et al. 2009). Central leptin gene therapy in the transgenic diabetic mice also imposed euglycemia (Ueno et al. 2006; Yoshioka et al. 1997). Akita mice are severely insulinopenic due to a dominant mutation in the Ins2 gene, and suffer from an early onset of hyperglycemia and diabetes mellitus (Ueno et al. 2006; Yoshioka et al. 1997). In addition to abrogation of hyperglycemia, central rAAV-lep treatment also enhanced insulin sensitivity and glucose tolerance, and augmented the rate of glucose disposal in these two type 1 diabetes paradigms (Ueno et al. 2006).

A single icv rAAV-lep injection also abolished hyperglycemia and diabetes mellitus for the lifetime in WT mice and rats fed high fat, and obese *ob/ob* mice (Boghossian et al. 2006; Kalra 2008a; Kalra and Kalra

2005; Ueno et al. 2004). In addition to conferring euglycemia, central leptin gene therapy simultaneously abolished hyperinsulinemia by suppressing episodic insulin release from pancreatic β-cells, and enhanced insulin sensitivity and the rate of glucose disposal. It became apparent that central leptin gene therapy corrected type 2 diabetes by a two-pronged action, by suppressing hyperinsulinemia through a neurally mediated restraint on insulin efflux from pancreatic β-cells and, independently enhancing glucose metabolism in the periphery (Boghossian et al. 2006; Kalra 2008a,b; Ueno et al. 2004). Cumulatively, these findings identify, for the first time, the therapeutic potential of central leptin gene therapy to ameliorate etiologically disparate type 1 and type 2 diabetes.

5 Cardiovascular Disease Risk

5.1 Systemic Inflammation

The effect of augmenting hypothalamic leptin signaling on cardiovascular disease risks was investigated by assessing low grade systemic inflammation and cardiomyopathy (Boghossian et al. 2007; Brownlee 2005; Dube et al. 2008; Kalra 2008a). Although it is well known that diabetes increases the risk of cardiovascular diseases, a strong causal relationship between chronic systemic low grade inflammation and increased risk of cardiovascular disease has recently been uncovered (Dube et al. 2008; Kalra 2008a: Olshansky et al. 2005). We observed that concomitant with suppression of adiposity the circulating levels of two markers of systemic low grade inflammation, the C-reactive protein (CRP) and interleukin-6 (Il-6) decreased markedly after an icv injection of rAAV-lep. Blood levels of CRP, released from hepatocytes under the transcriptional control of interleukins, including Il-6, were significantly elevated in obese *ob/ob* mice, but normalized in association with abrogation of fatty liver in response to increased leptin signaling in the hypothalamus (Boghossian et al. 2007; Dube et al. 2008). It is highly plausible that a direct neural link between leptin responsive hypothalamic targets and liver normally operates to restrain hepatic CRP efflux (Dube et al. 2008).

Circulating levels of Il-6, the other marker of low grade systemic inflammation, were also elevated, but fell dramatically to control range after leptin signaling was instituted in the hypothalamus of *ob/ob* mice (Dube et al. 2008). We suspect that this diminution in Il-6 levels is a consequence of depletion of adipose tissue, a major source of Il-6 (Dube et al. 2008; Kalra 2008a; Kalra and Kalra 2005). Furthermore, since Il-6 is implicated in amplifying the inflammatory cascade response of several acute-phase reactants, such as CRP, we propose that an outflow of leptin signaling from the hypothalamus along the descending neural pathways to adipocytes first reduces Il-6 release which, in turn, leads to a drop in CRP secretion from hepatocytes. It is obvious that leptin insufficiency in the hypothalamus augments the rate of fat deposition and the resultant morbid obesity culminates in systemic low grade inflammation and increased risks of cardiovascular diseases. Furthermore, these findings lead one to suggest that increased leptin supply to the hypothalamus has the potential to reliably alleviate these cardiovascular disease risks on a long-term basis.

5.2 Cardiomyopathy

Besides arteriosclerosis, deterioration in heart function due to oxidative stress and apoptotic myocyte cell death, are the manifestations of diabetic cardiomyopathy (Brownlee 2005; Fiordaliso et al. 2001; Malhotra et al. 2009; Migliaccio et al. 1999). Since central leptin gene therapy reversed hyperglycemia, even in the absence of circulating insulin (Malhotra et al. 2009), we recently observed that sustenance of euglycemia decelerated diabetic cardiomyopathy in Akita mice by contemporaneously decreasing the impact of oxidative stress and protecting the heart from increased apoptosis (Malhotra et al. 2009).

6 Bone Remodeling

Leptin deficient *ob/ob* mice display a mosaic of abnormalities in bone architecture, such as decreased bone length, decreased overall bone mass, but site-specific increases in cancellous bone volume (Hamrick et al. 2004; Iwaniec et al. 2007, 2009). Increased supply of leptin, either by systemic administration or by hypothalamic leptin gene therapy, decreased cancellous bone volume (Iwaniec et al. 2007, 2009). In addition, leptin gene therapy restored all measurements, i.e. increased femur length and total femur bone volume, decreased cancellous bone volume/tissue volume, trabecular numbers and trabecular thickness in distal femur and lumbar vertebrae and increased trabecular spacing. Thus, leptin gene therapy in *ob/ob* mice normalized cortical as well as cancellous bone volume to that in WT mice, a response that persisted for the 30 weeks duration of the experiment (Iwaniec et al. 2007, 2009).

For the first time a role of osteocalcin, an osteoblast-specific hormone, in correcting skeletal abnormalities by central leptin gene therapy in *ob/ob* mice and in facilitation of bone remodeling via bone formation in WT rodents, was recently reported (Kalra et al. 2009). Enhanced leptin signaling in the hypothalamus augmented circulating levels of osteocalcin in association with improved skeletal architecture (Iwaniec et al. 2007; Kalra et

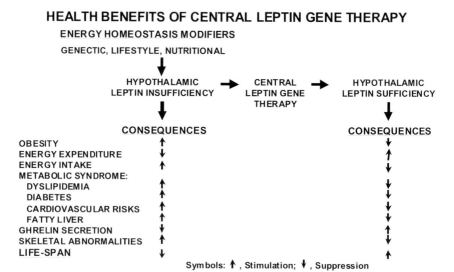

Figure 1

al. 2009). Seemingly, increased hypothalamic relay of information propagated by hypothalamic leptin receptors stimulates osteocalcin efflux from osteoblasts, a necessary step in bone remodeling for retention of normal skeletal phenotype (Iwaniec et al. 2007; Kalra et al. 2009).

7 Biomarkers of Aging and Life-span

That morbid obesity due to environmental and genetic causes invariably engenders a variety of life-threatening complications is well known (Fig. 1). According to clinical surveys (Kalra 2008a,b; Kalra and Kalra 2005; Olshansky et al. 2005), the disease cluster of metabolic syndrome, characterized by glucose intolerance, hyperglycemia, hyperinsulinemia, insulin resistance, hypertension, cardiovascular and renal failure and fatty liver disease, is a major risk factor for shortening life-span. Also, decreases in circulating ghrelin, a growth hormone secretagogue, and insulin-like growth factor-1, have been shown to be the endocrine biomarkers of early aging and mortality. Obese *ob/ob* mice, an example of monogenic obesity, display these biomarkers of aging and early mortality (Boghossian et al. 2006, 2007; Kalra 2008a). We observed that a single icv rAAV-lep injection more than doubled the life-span of *ob/ob* mice (Boghossian et al. 2007). Presumably, increased availability of optimal amounts of bioactive leptin within the hypothalamic targets, but insufficient to leak into cerebrospinal fluid for transfer into peripheral circulation, drastically reduced visceral fat, blood levels of glucose, insulin, and IGF-1 and augmented ghrelin levels (Fig. 1, Kalra 2008a; Kalra and Kalra 2005; Lecklin et al. 2005; Otukonyong et al. 2005a). Thus, introduction of ectopic leptin gene into the hypothalamus to ameliorate various life-threatening biomarkers for life-span extension is apparently a durable and safe therapy.

8 Concluding Remarks

Collectively, these findings affirm the hypothesis that it is possible to avert the onset of obesity and attendant disease cluster of metabolic syndrome, skeletal abnormalities, and early mortality by maintaining adequate leptin signaling in the hypothalamus (Fig. 1). Furthermore, bioavailability of leptin with gene therapy selectively in the hypothalamus is apparently safe and durable therapy to ameliorate type 1 and type 2 diabetes and normalize life-span. Therefore, we advocate clinical testing of central leptin gene therapy or of long-acting leptin mimetics to decelerate life-threatening pathophysiologic sequalae attending the worldwide epidemic of obesity and the metabolic syndrome.

Acknowledgment. Research summarized in this article was supported by grants from the National Institutes of Health (DK 37273).

References

Bagnasco M, MG Dube, et al. (2002) Evidence for the existence of distinct central appetite and energy expenditure pathways and stimulation of ghrelin as revealed by hypothalamic site-specific leptin gene therapy. Endocrinology 143(11): 4409-4421

Banks WA, CR DiPalma, et al. (1999) Impaired transport of leptin across the blood-brain barrier in obesity. Peptides 20(11): 1341-1345

Beretta E, MG. Dube, et al. (2002) Long-term suppression of weight gain, adiposity, and serum insulin by central leptin gene therapy in prepubertal rats: Effects on serum ghrelin and appetite-regulating genes. Ped. Res. 52: 189-198

Boghossian S, MG Dube, et al. (2006) Hypothalamic clamp on insulin release by leptin-transgene expression. Peptides 27(12): 3245-3254

Boghossian S, N Ueno, et al. (2007) Leptin gene transfer in the hypothalamus enhances longevity in adult monogenic mutant mice in the absence of circulating leptin. Neurobiol Aging 28(10): 1594-1604

Briley LP and LA Szczech (2006) Leptin and renal disease. Semin Dial 19(1): 54-59

Brownlee M (2005) The pathobiology of diabetic complications: a unifying mechanism. Diabetes 54: 1615-1625

Clark JT, PS Kalra, et al. (1984) Neuropeptide Y and human pancreatic polypeptide stimulate feeding behavior in rats. Endocrinology 115(1): 427-429

Correia MLG. and K Rahmouni (2006) Role of leptin in the cardiovascular and endocrine complications of metabolic syndrome. Diabetes, Obesity, and Metabolism 8(6): 603-610

Dhillon H, Y Ge, et al. (2000) Long-term differential modulation of genes encoding orexigenic and anorexigenic peptides by leptin delivered by rAAV vector in ob/ob mice. Relationship with body weight change. Regul Pept 92(1-3): 97-105

Dhillon H, SP Kalra, et al. (2001) Central leptin gene therapy suppresses body weight gain, adiposity and serum insulin without affecting food consumption in normal rats: A long-term study. Regul Pept 99(2-3): 69-77

Dube MG, SP Kalra, et al. (2007) Low abundance of NPY in the hypothalamus can produce hyperphagia and obesity. Peptides 28: 475-479

Dube MG, R Torto, et al. (2008) Increased leptin expression selectively in the hypothalamus suppresses inflammatory markers CRP and IL-6 in leptin-deficient diabetic obese mice. Peptides 29: 593-598

Fiordaliso F, A Leri, et al. (2001) Hyperglycemia activates p53 and p53 regulated genes leading to myocyte cell death. Diabetes 50: 2363-2375

Friedman JM and JL Halaas (1998) Leptin and the regulation of body weight in mammals. Nature 395(6704): 763-770

Hamrick MW, C Pennington, et al. (2004) Leptin deficiency produces contrasting phenotypes in bones of the limb and spine. Bone 34: 376-383

Hidaka S, H Yoshimatsu, et al. (2002) Chronic central leptin infusion restores hyperglycemia independent of food intake and insulin level in streptozotocin-induced diabetic rats. Faseb J 16(6): 509-518

Iwaniec UT, S Boghossian, et al. (2007) Central leptin gene therapy corrects skeletal abnormalities in leptin-deficient ob/ob mice. Peptides 28(5): 1012-9

Iwaniec UT, MG Dube, et al. (2009) Body mass influences cortical bone mass independent of leptin signaling. Bone 44: 404-412

Kalra SP (2008a) Central leptin insufficiency syndrome: An interactive etiology for obesity, metabolic and neural diseases and for designing new therapeutic interventions. Peptides 29: 127-138

Kalra SP (2008b) Disruption in the leptin-NPY link underlies the pandemic of diabetes and metabolic syndrome: New therapeutic approaches. Nutrition 24: 820-826

Kalra SP, M Bagnasco, et al. (2003) Rhythmic, reciprocal ghrelin and leptin signaling: new insight in the development of obesity. Regul Pept 111(1-3): 1-11

Kalra SP, MG Dube, et al. (2009) Leptin increases osteoblast-specific osteocalcin release through a hypothalamic relay. Peptides doi:10.1016/j.peptides.2009.01.020

Kalra SP, MG Dube, et al. (1999) Interacting appetite-regulating pathways in the hypothalamic regulation of body weight. Endocr Rev 20: 68-100

Kalra SP and PS Kalra (2005) Gene transfer technology: a preventive neurotherapy to curb obesity, ameliorate metabolic syndrome and extend life-expectancy. Trends Pharmacol Sci 26(10): 488-495

Kalra SP, N Ueno, et al. (2005) Stimulation of appetite by ghrelin is regulated by leptin restraint: peripheral and central sites of action. J Nutr 135(5): 1331-1335

Kastin AJ and W Pan (2006) Intranasal leptin: blood-brain barrier bypass (BBBB) for obesity? Endocrinology 147(5): 2086-2087

Kojima S, A Asakawa, et al. (2009) Central leptin gene therapy, a substitute for insulin therapy to ameliorate hyperglycemia and hyperphagia, and promote survival in insulin-deficient diabetic mice. Peptides doi:10.1016/j.peptides.2009.01.007

Lecklin AH, MG Dube, et al. (2005) Perigestational suppression of weight gain with central leptin gene therapy results in lower weight F1 generation. Peptides 26: 1176-1187

Malhotra A, H Vashistha, et al. (2009) Inhibition of p66ShcA redox activity in cardiac muscle cells attenuates hyperglycemia-induced oxidative stress and apoptosis. American Journal of Physiology-Heart and Circulatory Physiology 296: 380-388

Migliaccio E, M Giorgio, et al. (1999) The p66Shc adaptor protein controls oxidative stress and life span in mammals. Nature 402: 309-313

Olshansky SJ, DJ Passaro, et al. (2005) A potential decline in life expectancy in the United States in the 21st century. N Engl J Med 352(11): 1138-1145

Otukonyong EE, MG Dube, et al. (2005a) Central leptin differentially modulates ultradian secretory patterns of insulin, leptin and ghrelin independent of effects on food intake and body weight. Peptides 26(12): 2559-2566

Otukonyong EE, MG Dube, et al. (2005b) High fat diet-induced ultradian leptin and insulin hypersecretion and ghrelin is absent in obesity-resistant rats. Obesity Research 13: 991-999

Rigamonti AE, AI Pincelli, et al. (2002) Plasma ghrelin concentrations in elderly subjects: comparison with anorexic and obese patients. J Endocrinol 175(1): R1-R5

Ueno N, MG Dube, et al. (2004) Leptin modulates orexigenic effects of ghrelin and attenuates adiponectin and insulin levels and selectively the dark-phase feeding as revealed by central leptin gene therapy. Endocrinology 145(9): 4176-4184

Ueno N, A Inui, et al. (2006) Leptin transgene expression in the hypothalamus enforces euglycemia in diabetic, insulin-deficient nonobese Akita mice and leptin-deficient obese ob/ob mice. Peptides 27: 2332-2342

Yoshioka M, T Kayo, et al. (1997) A novel locus, Mody4, distal to D7Mit189 on chromosome 7 determines early-onset NIDDM in nonobese C57BL/6 (Akita) mutant mice. Diabetes 46(5): 887-894

Feeding regulation in the brain: Involvement of Neuropeptide W

Fumiko Takenoya[1,2], Haruaki Kageyama[1], Yukari Date[3], Masamitsu Nakazato[4], Seiji Shioda[1]

[1]Department of Anatomy I, Showa University School of Medicine, 1-5-8 Hatanodai, Shinagawa-ku, Tokyo 142-8555, Japan
<e-mail>haruaki@med.showa-u.ac.jp, shioda@med.showa-u.ac.jp
[2]Department of Physical Education, Hoshi University School of Pharmacy and Pharmaceutical Science, 2-4-41 Ebara, Shinagawa, Tokyo 142-8501, Japan
<e-mail>kuki@hoshi.ac.jp
[3]Department of Frontier Science Research Center, University of Miyazaki, 5200 Kiyotake, Miyazaki 889-1692, Japan
<e-mail> dateyuka@med.miyazaki-u.ac.jp
[4]Department of Division of Neurology, Respirology, Endocrinology, and Metabolism, Department of Internal Medicine, Faculty of Medicine, University of Miyazaki, 5200 Kiyotake, Miyazaki 889-1692, Japan
<e-mail>nakazato@med.miyazaki-u.ac.jp

Summary. Orphan G protein-coupled receptors (GPCRs) as targets to identify new transmitters have led over the last decade to the discovery of at least twelve novel neuropeptide families. Interestingly, several of these novel neuropeptides have physiological effects that include the modulation of food intake and energy expenditure. Neuropeptide W (NPW) is a novel neuropeptide which was recently isolated from the porcine hypothalamus and shown to be an endogenous ligand for the GPR7 and GPR8 orphan G protein-coupled receptors. NPW is widely distributed in the brain. Infusion of NPW is known to increase food intake in the light phase but inhibit intake in the dark phase. In spite of numerous morphological studies on NPW, its function has yet to be fully elucidated. Moreover, as the distribution of NPW-positive cell bodies in the hypothalamus has not been described, a detailed examination of NPW's distribution and localization in this brain region is required. The expression of NPW mRNA was demonstrated in the hypothalamic paraventricular nucleus (PVN), arcuate nucleus (ARC), ventromedial nucleus (VMH) and lateral hypothalamus (LH). NPW-like immunoreactivity (LI) was dramatically enhanced in animals pretreated with colchicine. At the light microscopic level, NPW-LI cell bodies have been identified in the preoptic areas (POA), PVN, ARC, VMH, LH, periaqueductal gray (PAG), lateral parabrachial nucleus (LPB) and prepositus nucleus. NPW-LI axon terminals have also been observed in the POA, bed nucleus of the stria terminals, amygdala, PVN, ARC, VMH, LH by electron microscopy. In addition, at the electron microscopic level, NPW-LI cell bodies and dendritic processes were often observed receiving inputs from other unknown neurons in the ARC, PVN, VMH and amygdala. Moreover, double immunostaining experiments showed that NPW-LI axon terminals were in close apposition to orexin-, MCH-, and NPY-containing neurons in the hypothalamus. These morphological and physiological findings strongly suggest that NPW participates in the regulation of feeding behavior in harmony with other feeding-regulating neurons in the hypothalamus.

Key words. Neuropeptide W (NPW), hypothalamus, feeding, neuronal network, Rat,

1 Introduction

It is well known that G protein-coupled receptors (GPCRs) form the largest family of membrane proteins that recognize extracellular messengers (Bockaert and Pin 1999). GPCRs are also known to mediate a variety of intracellular responses leading to the regulation of numerous physiological functions. GPCRs provide enormous potential for new drug development given that they are already the targets of nearly 50% of all prescription drugs including antihistamines, neuroleptics and antihypertensives (Howard et al. 2001). Interestingly, novel neuropeptides such as orexin, ghrelin, melanin-concentrating hormone (MCH), galanin-like peptide (GALP), neuropeptide B (NPB) and neuropeptide W (NPW) have had a strong impact on our understanding of the mechanisms that regulate obesity and energy homeostasis. In this chapter, I will focus on NPW, which is a newly identified GPCR ligand, and review its structure, function, distribution and localization in the brain.

2 NPW as a ligand for GPR7 and GPR8

O'Dowd and colleagues originally identified endogenous ligands of the GPCRs GPR7 and GPR8 that were originally identified by cloning the opioid somatostatin-like receptor genes from human genomic DNA (O'Dowd et al. 1995). GPR7 and GPR8 are thus quite closely related to opioid receptors. While GPR7 is found both in humans and rodents, GPR8 is apparently expressed only in humans (Lee et al. 1999). By using RT–PCR analysis, both GPR7 and GPR8 mRNA were detected at abundant levels in human tissues in the central nervous system (CNS) (Fujii et al. 2002). In particular, high levels of GPR7 mRNA were found in the hippocampus and amygdala (Brezillon et al. 2003). However, in the human brain, GPR7 and GPR8 mRNA is not found in many regions. On the other hand, in the rat, strong GPR7 mRNA expression was detected by RT–PCR analysis in the hypothalamus and amygdala (Fujii et al. 2002). In addition, *in situ* hybridization studies have revealed that GPR7 mRNA is present in the rat hypothalamus, including the ARC, VMH, PVN, dorsomedial nucleus (DMH) and supraoptic nucleus (SON) (Jackson et al. 2006; Lee et al. 1999). These nuclei in the hypothalamus are well known to be involved in feeding regulation and energy homeostasis. However, a detailed study to compare the distributions of both GPR7 and GPR8 in brain has not yet been done. It was reported that GPR7 mRNA is expressed in the hippocampus (Lee et al. 1999), but radio-ligand binding assays were unable to demonstrate the presence of its protein in this region (Singh et al. 2004).

3 Identification of neuropeptide W (NPW)

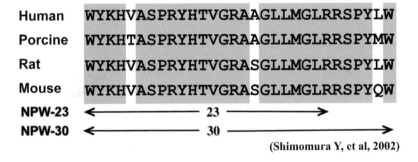

Fig.1. Amino acid sequences of NPW-23 and NPW-30. Shaded areas show similarities in amino acid sequence identities between human, porcine, rat and mouse.

The search for endogenous ligands for GPR7 or GPR8 led to the characterization of new peptides consisting of 23- and 30-amino acid residues (Fig.1). These neuropeptides, termed neuropeptide W-23 (NPW23) and neuropeptide W-30 (NPW30), were isolated from the porcine hypothalamus as endogenous ligands for GPR7 and GPR8 (Shimomura et al. 2002;Tanaka et al. 2003). NPW is named for tryptophan residues at the N and C termini of NPW30. Synthetic NPW23 and NPW30 were shown to bind and activate both GPR7 and GPR8 at similar effective doses (Shimomura et al. 2002; Tanaka et al. 2003). In *in vitro* experiments, human

NPW23 and NPW30 were shown to have a similar potency to activate human GPR7. NPW mRNA expression in the human CNS was strongest in the substantia nigra, amygdala and hippocampus (Fujii et al. 2002). In the mouse brain, NPW mRNA was not detected in the amygdala and hippocampus, whereas moderate expression was detected in the dorsal raphe nuclei (DRN), periaqueductal grey (PAG), and Edinger Westphal nuclei (EW). *In situ* hybridization studies have revealed NPW mRNA in the PAG, ventral tegmental area (VTA) and DRN in the mouse CNS (Tanaka et al. 2003), and in the PAG, EW and VTA in the rat brain (Kitamura et al. 2006).

4 Distribution of NPW in the brain

In immunohistochemical studies, we first tested the effect of colchicine treatment of animals prior to brain fixation. We demonstrated that NPW-LI was dramatically enhanced when animals were pre-treated with colchicine compared to untreated controls (Takenoya et al. 2008). Dan et al have already reported that NPW-LI was dramatically enhanced in colchicine-treated rats (Dun et al. 2003). They and we have reported that NPW-LI cell bodies are widely distributed in the brain, including the POA, PVN, SON, ARC, dorsal and lateral hypothalamic areas and anterior and posterior pituitary gland (Dun et al. 2003; Takenoya et al. 2008) (Fig.1). However, Kitamura et al. reported that NPW-LI cell bodies were identifiable in the PVN in rats and mice, but, for two separate reasons, this was probably due to non-specific staining. First, NPW-LI in the PVN is still observed in NPW gene-deficient mice when different commercially available antibodies are used. Second, NPW mRNA is not detected in the PVN of rats or mice by *in situ* hybridization (Hondo et al. 2008; Kitamura et al. 2006). In contrast, using RT-PCR, we identified NPW-LI cell bodies in the PVN as well as in the ARC, LH and VMH (data not shown). Recently, we observed NPW-LI axon terminals have also been observed in the POA, bed nucleus of the stria terminals (BST), amygdala, PVN, ARC, VMH, LH by electron microscopy. We also found that NPW-LI cell bodies were present in the EW, PAG, lateral parabrachial nucleus (LPB), medial parabrachial nucleus (MPB) in the rat brain as reported by Kitamura et al. (Kitamura et al. 2006).

In contrast, we observed NPW-LI processes in several other regions such as the lateral septum, BST, dorsomedial and posterior hypothalamus, central amygdaloid nucleus (Ce), hippocampus, interpeduncular nucleus, inferior colliculus, lateral parabrachial nucleus, facial nucleus and hypoglossal nucleus.

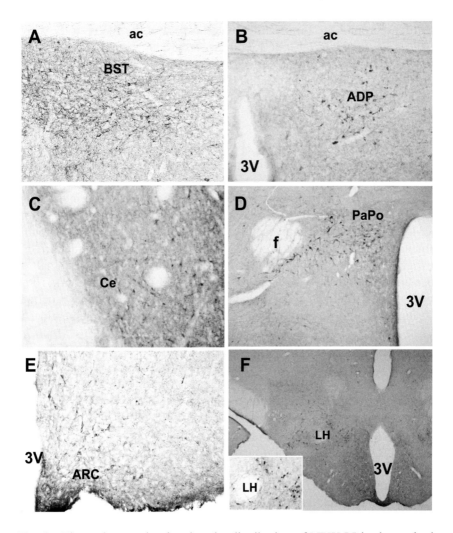

Fig. 2. Photomicrographs showing the distribution of NPW-LI in the rat brain. NPW-LI processes are seen in the bed nucleus of the stria terminalis (BST) (A), and the central amygdaloid nucleus (Ce)(C). NPW-LI cell bodies are seen in the anterodorsal preoptic nucleus (ADP)(B), posterior part (PaPo) of the paraventricular nucleus (D), arcuate nucleus (ARC)(E), and lateral hypothalamic area (LH)(F). ac: anterior commissure; f: fornix; 3V: 3rd ventricle.

In addition, we found that many NPW-LI processes could be observed in the central amygdaloid nucleus and BST (Fig2-A, C). Given the location of neurons with NPW-LI, these findings strongly suggest that NPW is involved in the emotive responses and regulation of reproduction in addition to feeding regulation. Interestingly, a high density of NPW-LI processes was found around the fornix in the anterior part of the LH region. At this level, very few NPW-LI cell bodies were detected. However, many NPW-LI cell bodies were observed in the region where the mammillary recess of the 3rd ventricle appears. NPW-LI cell bodies in the LH were thus observed within a narrow space in the caudal hypothalamus (Fig2-F). In addition, large numbers of neurons containing feeding regulating peptides such as orexin (Sakurai et al. 1998) and MCH (Kawauchi et al. 1983) have been shown to be present in the LH. We have also observed, at the electron microscopic level, NPW-LI cell bodies and dendritic processes were often observed receiving inputs from other unknown neurons in the ARC, PVN, VMH and amygdala (data not shown). In addition very close interactions between NPW-containing nerve processes and orexin- and MCH-containing neuronal cell bodies and processes by double immunostaining (Takenoya et al. 2008). Furthermore, we have identified at the light and electron microscope level, NPY-positive axon terminals in close apposition to NPW-LI neurons in the PVN (data not shown). These morphological findings suggest that NPW has neuromodulatory functions in feeding behavior in conjunction with other feeding regulating peptides in the brain.

5 Feeding regulation induced by NPW

In rat, GPR7 is expressed in the hypothalamus, including its feeding centers, suggesting it probably has a modulatory role for NPW in the control of feeding regulation. Some physiological studies have shown that the intracerebroventricular (icv) infusion of NPW affects food intake. For example, Shimomura et al. (Shimomura et al. 2002) reported that icv administration of NPW23 induced acute food in take on the light phase. On the other hand, in the dark phase, the icv infusion of NPW decreases food intake in the first 48 h (Mondal et al. 2003) even though the first 2 h following NPW injection is characterized by a hyperphagic state (Tanaka et al. 2003). GPR7 is expressed in the suprachiasmatic nucleus which is considered to control the circadian rhythm (Lee et al. 1999; Singh et al. 2004), hence the effect of the light/dark cycle in modulating NPW's action. It has also been suggested that chronic infusion of NPW reduces body weight and increases body temperature, heat production and oxygen consumption. Furthermore, by using GPR7 knockout mice, administration of NPW has hyperphagic and decreased energy expenditure effects. These results suggest that NPW is an anorexigenic peptide. It should be noted that these effects are evident in males but not on females, so the effects of NPW on energy balance may be sexually dimorphic (Ishii et al. 2003). In addition, icv infusion of NPW in rats initially provokes acute food intake (Mondal et al. 2003), while icv infusion of NPW in free-feeding rats suppresses feeding for an extended time (Shimomura et al. 2002).

Other reports have shown that administration of NPW increases c-Fos expression in the LH and PVN (Levine et al. 2005). These data suggest an appetite-regulating function of NPW in the hypothalamus and other brain regions. Interestingly, NPW is expressed in the stomach in addition to the CNS. The presence of NPW has been demonstrated in rat stomach antral cells and a decreased level of NPW has been reported in fasted animals; upon re-feeding, levels of NPW increase to normal in these animals (Mondal et al. 2006). NPW has been reported to lower blood leptin concentrations, with this mechanism possibly inferring the existence of an NPW-mediated regulation of energy homeostasis (Rucinski et al. 2007)

6 Acknowledgments

This work was supported in part by grants from the Ministry of Education, Science, Sports and Culture (T.F., H.K., S.S.), a High- technology Research Center Project from the Ministry of Education, Science, Sports and Culture of Japan (S.S.), and the CREST program of JST (S.S.).

7 References

Bockaert J, Pin JP (1999) Molecular tinkering of G protein-coupled receptors: an evolutionary success. EMBO J 18:1723-1729

Brezillon S, Lannoy V, Franssen JD, Le Poul E, Dupriez V, Lucchetti J, Detheux M, Parmentier M (2003) Identification of natural ligands for the orphan G protein-coupled receptors GPR7 and GPR8. J Biol Chem 278:776-783

Dun, SL, Brailoiu GC, Yang J, Chang JK, Dun NJ (2003) Neuropeptide W-immunoreactivity in the hypothalamus and pituitary of the rat. Neurosci Lett 349:71-74

Fujii R, Yoshida H, Fukusumi S, Habata Y, Hosoya M, Kawamata Y, Yano T, Hinuma S, Kitada C, Asami T, Mori M, Fujisawa Y, Fujino M (2002) Identification of a neuropeptide modified with bromine as an endogenous ligand for GPR7. J Biol Chem 277:34010-34016

Hondo M, Ishii M, Sakurai T (2008) The NPB/NPW neuropeptide system and its role in regulating energy homeostasis, pain, and emotion. Results Probl Cell Differ 46:239-256

Howard AD, McAllister G, Feighner SD, Liu Q, Nargund RP, Van der Ploeg LH, Patchett, AA (2001) Orphan G-protein-coupled receptors and natural ligand discovery. Trends Pharmacol Sci 22: 132-140

Ishii M, Fei H, Friedman JM (2003) Targeted disruption of GPR7, the endogenous receptor for neuropeptides B and W, leads to metabolic defects and adult-onset obesity. Proc Natl Acad Sci U S A 100:10540-10545

Jackson VR, Lin SH, Wang Z, Nothacker HP, Civelli O (2006) A study of the rat neuropeptide B/neuropeptide W system using in situ techniques. J Comp Neurol 497:367-383

Kawauchi H, Kawazoe I, Tsubokawa M, Kishida M, Baker BI (1983) Characterization of melanin-concentrating hormone in chum salmon pituitaries. Nature 305:321-323

Kitamura Y, Tanaka H, Motoike T, Ishii M, Williams SC, Yanagisawa M, Sakurai T (2006) Distribution of neuropeptide W immunoreactivity and mRNA in adult rat brain. Brain Res 1093: 123-134

Lee DK, Nguyen T, Porter CA, Cheng R, George SR, O'Dowd BF (1999) Two related G protein-coupled receptors: the distribution of GPR7 in rat brain and the absence of GPR8 in rodents. Brain Res Mol Brain Res 71:96-103

Levine AS, Winsky-Sommerer R, Huitron-Resendiz S, Grace MK, de Lecea L (2005) Injection of neuropeptide W into paraventricular nucleus of hypothalamus increases food intake. Am J Physiol Regul Integr Comp Physiol 288:1727-1732

Mondal MS, Yamaguchi H, Date Y, Shimbara T, Toshinai K, Shimomura Y, Mori M, Nakazato M (2003) A role for neuropeptide W in the regulation of feeding behavior. Endocrinology 144:4729-4733

Mondal MS, Yamaguchi H, Date Y, Toshinai K, Kawagoe T, Tsuruta T, Kageyama H, Kawamura Y, Shioda S, Shimomura Y, Mori M, Nakazato M (2006) Neuropeptide W is present in antral G cells of rat, mouse, and human stomach. J Endocrinol 188:49-57

O'Dowd BF, Scheideler MA, Nguyen T, Cheng R, Rasmussen JS, Marchese A, Zastawny R, Heng HH, Tsui LC, Shi X, et al (1995) The cloning and chromosomal mapping of two novel human opioid-somatostatin-like receptor genes, GPR7 and GPR8, expressed in discrete areas of the brain. Genomics 28:84-91

Rucinski M, Nowak KW, Chmielewska J, Ziolkowska A, Malendowicz LK (2007) Neuropeptide W exerts a potent suppressive effect on blood leptin and insulin concentrations in the rat. Int J Mol Med 19:401-405

Sakurai T, Amemiya A, Ishii M, Matsuzaki I, Chemelli RM, Tanaka H, Williams SC, Richardson JA, Kozlowski GP, Wilson S, Arch, JR, Buckingham, RE, Haynes AC, Carr SA, Annan RS, McNulty DE, Liu WS, Terrett JA, Elshourbagy NA, Bergsma DJ, Yanagisawa M (1998) Orexins and orexin receptors: a family of hypothalamic neuropeptides and G protein-coupled receptors that regulate feeding behavior. Cell 92:573-585

Shimomura Y, Harada M, Goto M, Sugo T, Matsumoto Y, Abe M, Watanabe T, Asami T, Kitada C, Mori M, Onda H, Fujino M (2002) Identification of neuropeptide W as the endogenous ligand for orphan G-protein-coupled receptors GPR7 and GPR8. J Biol Chem 277:35826-35832

Singh G, Maguire JJ, Kuc RE, Fidock M, Davenport AP (2004) Identification and cellular localisation of NPW1 (GPR7) receptors for the novel neuropeptide W-23 by [125I]-NPW radioligand binding and immunocytochemistry. Brain Res 1017:222-226

Takenoya F, Kitamura S, Kageyama H, Nonaka N, Seki M, Itabashi K, Date Y, Nakazato M, Shioda S (2008) Neuronal interactions between neuropeptide W- and orexin- or melanin-concentrating hormone-containing neurons in the rat hypothalamus. Regul Pept 145:159-164

Tanaka H, Yoshida T, Miyamoto N, Motoike T, Kurosu H, Shibata K, Yamanaka A, Williams SC, Richardson JA, Tsujino N, Garry MG., Lerner MR, King DS, O'Dowd BF, Sakurai T, Yanagisawa M, (2003) Characterization of a family of endogenous neuropeptide ligands for the G protein-coupled receptors GPR7 and GPR8. Proc Natl Acad Sci U S A 100:6251-6256

Feeding regulation in the brain: Role of galanin-like peptide (GALP)

Haruaki Kageyama[1], Fumiko Takenoya[1,2], and Seiji Shioda[1]

[1]Department of Anatomy I, Showa University School of Medicine, 1-5-8 Hatanodai, Shinagawa-ku, Tokyo 142-8555, Japan
<e-mail>haruaki@med.showa-u.ac.jp, shioda@med.showa-u.ac.jp
[2]Department of Physical Education, Hoshi University School of Pharmacy and Pharmaceutical Science, 2-4-41 Ebara, Shinagawa, Tokyo 142-8501, Japan
<e-mail>kuki@hoshi.ac.jp

Summary. Galanin-like peptide (GALP), a 60-amino acid peptide that influences feeding behavior and energy metabolism, is produced in the hypothalamic arcuate nucleus (ARC). GALP-containing neurons send outputs to orexin-, melanin-concentrating hormone (MCH)-, and tyrosine hydroxylase (TH)-containing neurons, and receive inputs from orexin- and neuropeptide Y-containing neurons. In addition, some GALP-containing neurons have been shown to co-localize with α-melanocyte-stimulating hormone (α-MSH), which is an anorexigenic peptide derived from proopiomelanocortin (POMC). c-Fos experiments have shown that GALP activates neurons in the lateral hypothalamus (LH), a feeding center where orexin- and MCH-containing neurons are known to be located. Moreover, c-Fos expressions have been observed in orexin- but not MCH-containing neurons in the LH. To determine whether GALP regulates feeding behavior via orexin neurons, the feeding behavior of rats was studied following the intracerebroventricular (icv) injection of GALP with or without anti-orexin A and B immunoglobulin (IgG) pretreatment. The anti-orexin IgGs markedly inhibited GALP-induced acute hyperphagia. These results strongly suggest that orexin-containing neurons in the LH are targeted by GALP, and that GALP induces feeding activity through orexin-containing neurons in the LH. To clarify the neural network and the function of GALP neurons, we have generated a transgenic mouse strain which expresses enhanced green fluorescence protein (eGFP) under the control of a promoter of the GALP gene. Using confocal laser microscopy techniques, eGFP fluorescence was detected in the ARC of colchicine-treated GALP-eGFP transgenic mice. These transgenic animals could serve as a powerful tool in the morphological and electrophysiological analysis of GALP-containing neurons.

Key words. hypothalamus, neuropeptide, transgenic mouse, green fluorescent protein

1 Introduction

Galanin-like peptide (GALP) is 60 amino acid peptide which was discovered in porcine hypothalamus extracts using a binding assay for galanin receptors (Ohtaki et al. 1999). This peptide shares amino acid sequence homology with galanin (1-13) in position 9-21. The intracerebroventricular (icv) injection of GALP increases food intake in rats in the first 2 h after injection, but does not alter food intake in mice 2 h after injection (Krasnow et al. 2003; Lawrence et al. 2003; Matsumoto et al. 2002). However, in both species GALP decreases food intake and body weight gain 24 h after injection (Krasnow et al. 2003; Lawrence et al. 2002; Lawrence et al. 2003). These results suggest that GALP influences feeding behavior and energy metabolism in rodents.

2 Neuronal circuits involving GALP in the hypothalamus

GALP mRNA is expressed in the hypothalamic arcuate nucleus (ARC) of rodents (Fujiwara et al. 2002; Jureus et al. 2000; Kerr et al. 2000; Larm and Gundlach 2000; Shen and Gundlach 2004; Takatsu et al. 2001). The intraperitoneal injection of leptin increases the expression of GALP mRNA, which contrasts with the fasted state in which low plasma levels of leptin parallel that of decreased GALP mRNA expression. It has been demonstrated immunohistochemically that GALP-containing cell bodies are present in the ARC, and that more than 85% of GALP-containing neurons express leptin receptors on their surface membranes (Takatsu et al. 2001). These results suggest that the expression of GALP is controlled by leptin.

We have determined immunohistochemically some aspects of neuronal circuits involving GALP. GALP-containing fibers are present in several regions: the lateral hypothalamus (LH), the paraventricular nucleus (PVN), the bed nucleus of the stria terminalis (BST) and the medial preoptic area (MPA) (Takatsu et al. 2001; Takenoya et al. 2006; Takenoya et al. 2005). GALP-containing neurons send outputs to orexin- and melanin-concentrating hormone (MCH) in the LH, as well as tyrosine hydoxylase-containing neurons in the ARC (Kageyama et al. 2008; Takenoya et al. 2005). GALP-containing neurons receive inputs from orexin-containing neurons in the LH and from neuropeptide Y-containing neurons in the ARC

(Takenoya et al. 2003; Takenoya et al. 2002). GALP-containing neurons co-localize with α-melanin stimulating hormone (α-MSH), which is derived from proopiomelanocoltin (POMC) (Fig.1) (Takenoya et al. 2002). Furthermore, GALP-containing neurons also express orexin receptors (Takenoya et al. 2003). On this basis, it can be seen that GALP-containing neurons form neural circuits that involve several types of feeding-regulating peptide-containing neurons.

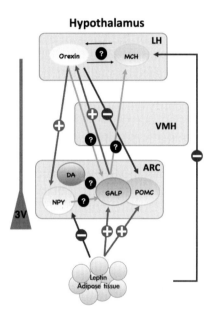

Fig. 1. Neuronal circuits involving GALP in the hypothalamic region. MCH, melanin-concentrating hormone; DA, dopamine; NPY, neuropeptide Y; POMC, proopiomelanocortin; LH, lateral hypothalamus, VMH, ventromedial hypothalamus; ARC, arcuate nucleus; 3V, third ventricle; +, physiological stimulating action; -, physiological suppressing action; ?, unknown.

3 Neuronal feeding-regulating pathways involving GALP

Icv injection of GALP activates many neuronal nuclei in the rat hypothalamus. The nuclei of neurons activated by GALP can be identified by their c-Fos expression, a marker of a neuronal activation, after central injection of GALP (Cunningham 2004; Fraley et al. 2003; Fraley et al. 2004; Kageyama et al. 2006; Kauffman et al. 2005; Kuramochi et al. 2006; Lawrence et al. 2003; Man and Lawrence 2008; Matsumoto et al. 2001). When GALP is injected into the lateral ventricle of the rat brain, c-Fos-like immunoreactivity can be identified in neurons located in the MPA, PVN, LH, ARC, supraoptic nucleus (SON) and dorsomedial nucleus of the hypothalamus (DMH), and the nucleus tractus solitarius in the brainstem (NTS) (Lawrence et al. 2003). Furthermore, GALP activates astrocytes but not microglia in the hypothalamus (Lawrence et al. 2003), and ependymal cells in the peri-third ventricle. However, c-Fos expression was hardly induced in the ventromedial hypothalamus. The exact location(s) of the main target area(s) of GALP in the brain or the kinds of cells affected in cases of increased food intake activity are yet to be fully identified.

The LH is a recognized feeding-regulation center in the rat brain, and GALP has been shown to induce c-Fos expression in many neurons within this region. In order to identify the nature of c-Fos-expressing neurons in the LH, we focused on orexin- and MCH-containing neurons, and performed double immunostaining for both c-Fos and orexin or MCH. c-Fos-like immunoreactivity was found to be observed in many orexin-immunopositive but not in MCH-immunopositive neurons in the LH (Kageyama et al. 2006). We also made a quantitative analysis of c-Fos expression in neurons in the LH after icv infusion of GALP. The number of c-Fos-immunopositive neurons in the GALP-infused group was more than twice that of the control group. In orexin-immunopositive neurons, the number of neurons showing c-Fos-like immunoreactivity more than doubled after infusion of GALP (Kageyama et al. 2006). These morphological observations suggest that GALP simulates orexin neurons but has no effect on MCH-immunopositive neurons. Furthermore, at the EM level, double-labeling immunohistochemistry experiments showed that GALP immunopositive axon terminals make synaptic contacts with orexin immunopositive cell bodies and their dendritic processes.

Although we have shown morphologically that GALP stimulates feeding behavior through orexin-containing neurons, it is not known whether endogenous orexin itself plays an important role in GALP-related feeding regulation. In order to determine whether GALP physiologically regulates feeding behavior via orexin-containing neurons, the feeding behavior of rats was studied following icv injection of GALP with or without anti-orexin A and B immunoglobulin (IgG) pretreatment. The anti-orexin IgGs markedly inhibited GALP-induced hyperphagia (Kageyama et al. 2006). These results suggest that orexin-containing neurons in the LH are targeted by GALP, and that GALP simulates feeding behavior through orexin-containing neurons in this brain region. Moreover, Kuramochi et al. (Kuramochi et al. 2006) reported that GALP activates NPY-containing neurons in the DMH and that this promotes feeding behavior. Thus, it is suggested that GALP mediates feeding behavior via 2 different pathways.

4 Generation of a transgenic mouse that expresses enhanced green fluorescent protein (eGFP) under the control of the GALP gene promoter

We attempted to visualize the neural circuitry involving GALP neurons and to clarify the function of GALP neurons using electrophysiological techniques such as patch clamp or intracellular calcium imaging experiments. In order to visualize GALP neurons without immunohistochemistry using anti-GALP antibody and to isolate GALP neurons for electrophysiological studies, we have generated a transgenic mouse that expresses enhanced green fluorescent protein (eGFP) under the control of the GALP gene promoter. We constructed a transgene in which a 12.6 kb of DNA fragment containing presumed regulatory region of mouse GALP was ligated to a fragment containing both cDNA encoding eGFP and a poly adenylate signal site of the rabbit beta-globin gene. Transgenic mice were generated by microinjection of the transgene into fertilized eggs. eGFP fluoresces in the ARC of colchicine-treated GALP-eGFP transgenic mice as visualized using confocal laser microscopy. The results were consistent with other studies showing that GALP is located in the hypothalamic ARC. These transgenic animals could serve as a powerful tool for the morphological and electrophysiological analysis of GALP-containing neurons.

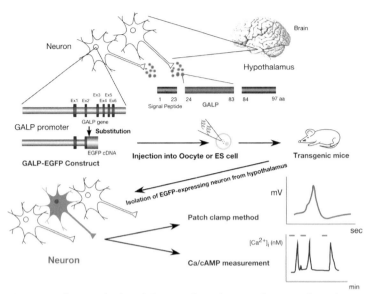

Fig. 2. Strategy for analysis of GALP function. Refer to color plates.

5 Acknowledgments

The authors thank Dr. Tetsuya Ohtaki of Takeda Chemical Industrial Company, Dr. Koji Toshinai, Prof. Yukari Date and Prof. Masamitsu Nakazato of Miyazaki University, and Ms. Sachi Kato of Showa University for their help in carrying out this work. This study was supported in part by a Grant-in-Aid for Scientific Research "KAKENHI" from the Ministry of Education, Culture, Sports, Science and Technology of Japan (#19659047, # 19590196).

6 References

Cunningham MJ (2004). Galanin-like peptide as a link between metabolism and reproduction. J Neuroendocrinol 16:717-723.

Fraley GS, Shimada I, Baumgartner JW, Clifton DK, and Steiner RA (2003). Differential patterns of Fos induction in the hypothalamus of the rat following central injections of galanin-like peptide and galanin. Endocrinology 144:1143-1146.

Fraley GS, Thomas-Smith SE, Acohido BV, Steiner RA, and Clifton DK (2004). Stimulation of sexual behavior in the male rat by galanin-like peptide. Horm Behav 46:551-557.

Fujiwara K, Adachi S, Usui K, Maruyama M, Matsumoto H, Ohtaki T, Kitada C, Onda H, Fujino M, and Inoue K (2002). Immunocytochemical localization of a galanin-like peptide (GALP) in pituicytes of the rat posterior pituitary gland. Neurosci Lett 317:65-68.

Jureus A, Cunningham MJ, McClain ME, Clifton DK, and Steiner RA (2000). Galanin-like peptide (GALP) is a target for regulation by leptin in the hypothalamus of the rat. Endocrinology 141:2703-2706.

Kageyama H, Kita T, Toshinai K, Guan JL, Date Y, Takenoya F, Kato S, Matsumoto H, Ohtaki T, Nakazato M, and Shioda S (2006). Galanin-like peptide promotes feeding behaviour via activation of orexinergic neurons in the rat lateral hypothalamus. J Neuroendocrinol 18:33-41.

Kageyama H, Takenoya F, Hori Y, Yoshida T, and Shioda S (2008). Morphological interaction between galanin-like peptide- and dopamine-containing neurons in the rat arcuate nucleus. Regul Pept 145:165-168.

Kauffman AS, Buenzle J, Fraley GS, and Rissman EF (2005). Effects of galanin-like peptide (GALP) on locomotion, reproduction, and body weight in female and male mice. Horm Behav 48:141-151.

Kerr NC, Holmes FE, and Wynick D (2000). Galanin-like peptide (GALP) is expressed in rat hypothalamus and pituitary, but not in DRG. Neuroreport 11:3909-3913.

Krasnow SM, Fraley GS, Schuh SM, Baumgartner JW, Clifton DK, and Steiner RA (2003). A role for galanin-like peptide in the integration of feeding, body weight regulation, and reproduction in the mouse. Endocrinology 144:813-822.

Kuramochi M, Onaka T, Kohno D, Kato S, and Yada T (2006). Galanin-like peptide stimulates food intake via activation of neuropeptide Y neurons in the hypothalamic dorsomedial nucleus of the rat. Endocrinology 147:1744-1752.

Larm JA, and Gundlach AL (2000). Galanin-like peptide (GALP) mRNA expression is restricted to arcuate nucleus of hypothalamus in adult male rat brain. Neuroendocrinology 72:67-71.

Lawrence CB, Baudoin FM, and Luckman SM (2002). Centrally administered galanin-like peptide modifies food intake in the rat: a comparison with galanin. J Neuroendocrinol 14:853-860.

Lawrence CB, Williams T, and Luckman SM (2003). Intracerebroventricular galanin-like peptide induces different brain activation compared with galanin. Endocrinology 144:3977-3984.

Man PS, and Lawrence CB (2008). The effects of galanin-like peptide on energy balance, body temperature and brain activity in the mouse and rat are independent of the GALR2/3 receptor. J Neuroendocrinol 20:128-137.

Matsumoto H, Noguchi J, Takatsu Y, Horikoshi Y, Kumano S, Ohtaki T, Kitada C, Itoh T, Onda H, Nishimura O, and Fujino M (2001). Stimulation effect of galanin-like peptide (GALP) on luteinizing hormone-releasing hormone-mediated luteinizing hormone (LH) secretion in male rats. Endocrinology 142:3693-3696.

Matsumoto Y, Watanabe T, Adachi Y, Itoh T, Ohtaki T, Onda H, Kurokawa T, Nishimura O, and Fujino M (2002). Galanin-like peptide stimulates food intake in the rat. Neurosci Lett 322:67-69.

Ohtaki T, Kumano S, Ishibashi Y, Ogi K, Matsui H, Harada M, Kitada C, Kurokawa T, Onda H, and Fujino M (1999). Isolation and cDNA cloning of a novel galanin-like peptide (GALP) from porcine hypothalamus. J Biol Chem 274:37041-37045.

Shen J, and Gundlach AL (2004). Galanin-like peptide mRNA alterations in arcuate nucleus and neural lobe of streptozotocin-diabetic and obese zucker rats. Further evidence for leptin-dependent and independent regulation. Neuroendocrinology 79:327-337.

Takatsu Y, Matsumoto H, Ohtaki T, Kumano S, Kitada C, Onda H, Nishimura O, and Fujino M (2001). Distribution of galanin-like peptide in the rat brain. Endocrinology 142:1626-1634.

Takenoya F, Aihara K, Funahashi H, Matsumoto H, Ohtaki T, Tsurugano S, Yamada S, Katoh S, Kageyama H, Takeuchi M, and Shioda S (2003). Galanin-like peptide is target for regulation by orexin in the rat hypothalamus. Neurosci Lett 340:209-212.

Takenoya F, Funahashi H, Matsumoto H, Ohtaki T, Katoh S, Kageyama H, Suzuki R, Takeuchi M, and Shioda S (2002). Galanin-like peptide is co-localized with alpha-melanocyte stimulating hormone but not with neuropeptide Y in the rat brain. Neurosci Lett 331:119-122.

Takenoya F, Guan JL, Kato M, Sakuma Y, Kintaka Y, Kitamura Y, Kitamura S, Okuda H, Takeuchi M, Kageyama H, and Shioda S (2006). Neural interaction between galanin-like peptide (GALP)- and luteinizing hormone-releasing hormone (LHRH)-containing neurons. Peptides 27:2885-2893.

Takenoya F, Hirayama M, Kageyama H, Funahashi H, Kita T, Matsumoto H, Ohtaki T, Katoh S, Takeuchi M, and Shioda S (2005). Neuronal interactions between galanin-like-peptide- and orexin- or melanin-concentrating hormone-containing neurons. Regul Pept 126:79-83.

Neuropeptides, Bioamines, and Clinical Implications

Neuropeptide Y and its Role in Anxiety-related Disorders

Yvan Dumont[1], Julio César Morales-Medina[2], Rémi Quirion[3]

[1]Douglas Mental Health University Institute, 6875 LaSalle Boulevard, Montreal, QC, Canada, H4H 1R3
yvan.dumont@douglas.mcgill.ca
[2]Douglas Mental Health University Institute, Department of Neurology and Neurosurgery, McGill University, 6875 LaSalle Boulevard, Montreal, QC, Canada, H4H 1R3
julio.morales@douglas.mcgill.ca
[3]Douglas Mental Health University Institute, Department of Psychiatry, McGill University, 6875 LaSalle Boulevard, Montreal, QC, Canada, H4H 1R3
remi.quirion@douglas.mcgill.ca

Summary: Neuropeptide Y (NPY) is one of the most abundant peptide in the brain and has been implicated in various biological functions. Preclinical and clinical investigations have suggested that NPY, acting on specific receptors, has direct role in several psychiatric disorders, including depression and anxiety-related illnesses, which will be reviewed in this chapter. Increasing support for a role for NPY in mood disorders has been obtained over the past few years. The Y_1, Y_2 and Y_4 receptor subtypes have been particularly involved in these behaviours. For example, we reported that NPY Y_2 knockout mice display anxiolytic-like phenotype as assessed in the elevated plus maze and open field tests, suggesting a role of this receptor subtype in anxiety-related behaviours. Moreover, NPY Y_2 knockout mice display memory retention deficits as evaluated in the Morris water maze and object recognition tests, while acquisition performance, swim speed and visible platform performance were not significantly different between knockout and wild-type mice. Additionally, young and old rats overexpressing NPY were found to be resistant to acute physical restrain stress, but rather surprisingly, no memory deficit was observed in old transgenic rats, contrasting with data obtained in young transgenic animals. Aged NPY transgenic rats and NPY Y_2 knockout mice exhibit anxiolytic-like phenotypes, in accordance with results observed in younger animals. Interestingly, the ontogeny of various NPY receptor subtypes suggest further that they may be implicated in the etiology of anxiety-like phenotype observed in maternally deprived animals as important changes in NPY receptor distribution and levels occur during this critical period, especially for the Y_2 receptor subtype. Taken together, these results support the hypothesis that NPY and its receptors may be involved in the regulation of anxiety-related behaviours and provide evidence that this neuropeptide family is an attractive drug development target for these disorders.

Key words: Anxiety, Neuropeptide Y, Behavioural tests, Sedation, Ontogeny

1 Introduction

Anxiety is an emotion that reflects a state of cognitive and behavioural preparedness that an organism mobilizes in response to a potential threat. There are in fact two forms of anxieties, the non-pathological and the pathological one. The non-pathological form includes ``state anxiety'', which is an acute adaptive response of heightened vigilance and arousal and ``trait anxiety'', a measure of an individual's baseline reactivity or tendency to generate anxious response (Leonardo and Hen 2008). Pathological anxiety conditions include panic disorder, post-traumatic stress disorder (PTSD), generalized anxiety disorder (GAD), social anxiety disorder (SAD) or agoraphobia, obsessive-compulsive disorder (OCD), and specific phobias (Leonardo and Hen 2008; Mathew et al. 2008). Symptoms are manifested at the psychological, behavioural and physiological levels, and are thought to involve both endogenous predisposing factors (mostly genetic) and the ability of coping with stress (McEwen 2000; Southwick et al. 2005). These disorders are often associated with serious disabilities, increased rate of chronic medical conditions, and high level of comorbidity and overlap with a variety of neuropsychiatric conditions, such as depression and substance abuse (Mathew et al. 2008).

Current therapeutic strategies for the treatment of anxiety disorders include benzodiazepines, tricyclic antidepressants, monoamine oxidase A inhibitors, as well as monoamine uptake inhibitors (Nemeroff 2003). However, currently available anxiolytics possess various adverse side-effects including nausea, sexual dysfunction, anorexia, sweating, asthenia and tremor (Mathew et al. 2008). Additionally, the tolerability of benzodiazepine anxiolytics is reduced by sedation, cognitive impairments and dependence (Mathew et al. 2008). These observations have given rise to a search for alternative therapeutic targets for the treatment of anxiety-related disorders. In that regard, several neuropeptides have been suggested as potential alternatives including cholecystokinin, corticotrophin releasing factor (CRF), tachykinins and neuropeptide Y (Griebel 1999; Millan 2003). Data obtained using pharmacological or molecular tools as well as studies in human have consistently suggested a role for neuropeptide Y and its receptors in anxiety-related disorders.

Neuropeptide Y (NPY) is a 36 amino acid residues polypeptide isolated from porcine brain more than twenty five years ago (Tatemoto 1982). It belongs to a peptide family called the Y family, which includes peptide YY (PYY) and pancreatic polypeptides (PP). NPY is one of the most abundant brain peptides and is expressed in numerous regions where it is often colocalized with either noradrenaline, glutamate, GABA, somatostatin or the agouti-related protein (Kask et al. 2002). NPY is also one of the most highly conserved peptides from an evolutionary perspective (Larhammar 1996). Early studies have demonstrated that NPY is implicated in a broad range of biological effects including increased food and water intake (Stanley and Leibowitz 1984), facilitated learning and memory processes (Flood et al. 1987), inhibited glutamatergic and noradrenergic synaptic transmission (Colmers et al. 1987; Wahlestedt and Hakanson 1986), as well as GABAergic activity (Acuna-Goycolea et al. 2005; Kash and Winder 2006), affected locomotor behaviours (Ekman et al. 1986), hypothermia (Esteban et al. 1989), decreased sexual behaviours (Clark et al. 1985), altered cardiorespiratory parameters (Edvinsson et al. 1984; Harfstrand 1986), shifts in circadian rhythms (Albers and Ferris 1984), regulated release of luteinizing hormone releasing hormone (LHRH) (Kalra and Crowley 1984) and induced release of corticotrophin releasing factor (CRF) (Tsagarakis et al. 1989). It has also been shown that NPY can induce anxiolytic-like (Heilig et al. 1993) and antidepressant-like (Redrobe et al. 2002a) effects, in addition to a role in alcohol consumption (Thiele et al. 1998), epilepsy (Klapstein and Colmers 1997; Vezzani et al. 1999) and pain processes (Wang et al. 2000). Several of these effects appear to be physiologically relevant, based on data obtained using pharmacological approches, knockout mice or transgenic animals (for review see: Blomqvist and Herzog 1997; Carvajal et al. 2006b; Carvajal et al. 2007; Dumont et al. 2000b; Inui 2000; Kalra and Kalra 2006; Kask et al. 2002; Lin et al. 2004; Redrobe et al. 2002b; Vezzani et al. 1999).

Table 1. Agonists and antagonists of the NPY family

NPY receptor subtype	Agonists with nM affinities	Antagonists with nM affinities
Y_1	NPY PYY [Leu^{31}, Pro^{34}]NPY [Leu^{31}, Pro^{34}]PYY [Arg^6, Pro^{34}]NPY [Phe^7, Pro^{34}]NPY [D-His^{26}]NPY	BIBP3226 BIBO3304 GR231118 LY35789 J-104870 GI264879A J-115814 H409/22
Y_2	NPY PYY NPY3–36 PYY3–36 Truncated NPY C2-NPY	BIIE0246 JNJ-520778
Y_4	Rat PP Human PP GR231118 [Leu^{31}, Pro^{34}]PYY	none
Y_5	NPY PYY NPY3–36 PYY3–36 [Leu^{31}, Pro^{34}]NPY [Leu^{31}, Pro^{34}]PYY [hPP1–17, Ala^{31}, Aib^{32}]NPY [cPP1–7, NPY19–23, Ala^{31}, Aib^{32}, Gln^{34}]hPP Human PP	CGP71683A JCF109 NPY5RA GW438014A L-152,804

The various physiological functions of NPY are mediated by the activation of at least five receptor subtypes designated as Y_1, Y_2, Y_4, Y_5 and y_6 receptors (Michel et al. 1998). These receptors have been cloned and belong to the G-protein coupled receptor superfamily (Dumont et al. 2002). Each NPY receptor subtype exhibits a distinctive pharmacological profile (Table 1). To date, selective antagonists have been developed for the Y_1, Y_2 and Y_5, but not Y_4, receptor subtypes (Table 1). In the central nervous system, Y_1 and Y_2 receptors are broadly distributed, while Y_4 and Y_5 subtypes have a more restricted localization and are expressed at lower amounts (Dumont et al. 1998b; Dumont et al. 2000c; Dumont et al. 2004). The y_6 receptor subtype is only expressed in few species such as the mouse, dog and rabbit, and is a pseudogene in primates and human; it is not expressed in the rat (Michel et al. 1998).

2 Tests used to measure anxious-like behaviours

Fear and anxiety could be defined as the response of a subject to real or potential threats that may impair its homeostasis. This response may include physiological (increase in hearth rate, blood pressure, cortisol levels etc.) as well as behavioural (inhibition of ongoing behaviours, scanning, avoidance of the source of danger etc.) parameters. Anxiety-like behaviours in rodents have been mostly studied using few well established tests such as the elevated plus-maze, light/dark box and open-field tests. These procedures are based upon the exposure of subjects to unfamiliar, aversive places. However, it is now evident that anxiety is not a unitary phenomenon but could be divided in various forms including 'state' and 'trait' anxieties as well as 'normal' and 'pathological' anxieties. These various forms have been shown to be differently sensitive to various pharmacological challenges. Therefore, when measuring anxiety in animals, it is useful to have information on the type of anxiety processes involved in a given test (Belzung and Griebel 2001). Over 30 models are used in preclinical anxiety research and although some are based on physiological responses and others on drug-induced states, the vast majority employs "behavioural" approaches. The type of behaviour studied, however, varies considerably with the most obvious distinction being tests based on conditioned responses (Geller-Seifter, Vogel-punished and Fear-potentiated startle tests), versus those involving unconditioned behaviours (open field, elevated plus maze, light-dark box and social interaction tests). See a detailed review by File (2004) for a descriptions of these tests.

3 NPY and anxiety

3.1 Exogenous effects of NPY in behavioural tests

NPY, when administered intracerebroventricularly (icv) or into specific brain regions, induces anxiolytic activity in various behavioural tests widely used for the screening of anxiolytic compounds. NPY is reported to

Table 2. Effects of administered NPY on anxiety-related behaviours

Model	Treatment	Effect	Reference
Elevated plus maze	NPY	anxiolytic	1, 2, 3
	PYY	anxiolytic	4
	[Leu^{31}, Pro^{34}]PYY (Y$_1$)	anxiolytic	4, 5
	NPY2-36	anxiolytic	4
	NPY3-36 (Y$_2$)		6
	NPY13-36 (Y$_2$)	no effect	1, 5
	NPY13-36	anxiogenic	5
	BIBP3226 (Y$_1$)	anxiogenic	6
Open field	NPY	anxiolytic	2, 3
	[D-His^{26}]NPY (Y$_1$)	anxiolytic	3
	C2-NPY (Y$_2$)	no effect	3
Light-dark box	NPY	anxiolytic	2, 7
Social interaction	NPY	anxiolytic	8, 9
Vogel conflict	NPY	anxiolytic	1
	NPY13-36	no effect	1
Geller-Seifter	NPY	anxiolytic	10, 11
	[Leu^{31},Pro^{34}]NPY (Y$_1$)	anxiolytic	10, 12
	NPY13-36 (Y$_2$)	no effect	10,12
	[Gly^6, Glu^{26},Lys^{26},Pro^{34}]-NPY	anxiolytic	10
	PP	no effect	10
	PYY	anxiolytic	10
Fear-potentiated Startle	NPY	anxiolytic	2
	[Leu^{31},Pro^{34}]NPY	anxiolytic	4
	NPY 13-36 (Y$_2$)	no effect	4

Reference
1, Heilig et al. 1989a; 2, Karlsson et al. 2005; 3, Sorensen et al. 2004; 4, Broqua et al. 1995; 5, Nakajima et al. 1998; 6, Kask et al. 1996; 7, Pich et al. 1993; 8, Kask et al. 2001; 9, Sajdyk et al. 1999; 10, Britton et al. 1997; 11, Heilig et al. 1992; 12, Heilig et al. 1993

elicit anxiolytic-like effects in models of anxiety including exploratory behaviour-based tests such as the open field, elevated plus-maze, light-dark compartment test, social interaction, punished responding tests including Geller-Seifter test, Vogel-punished drinking test and fear-potentiated startle (See Table 2). Furthermore, using agonists and antagonists of the NPY family, it has been shown that the anxiolytic-like effects of NPY are mediated by the NPY Y_1 receptors (Britton et al. 1997; Broqua et al. 1995; Heilig et al. 1992; Nakajima et al. 1998; Sajdyk et al. 1999). Additionally, antisense inhibition of the NPY Y_1 receptor expression produced anxiogenic-like effects (Wahlestedt et al. 1993) and blocked the anxiolytic-like effects of NPY (Heilig 1995). However, as seen for traditional anxiolytics, sedative effects and suppressed locomotor activity have also been reported for NPY (Heilig et al. 1989a; Heilig and Murison 1987; Karlsson et al. 2005; Naveilhan et al. 2001), but these effects usually occur at higher doses. Overall, the robust anxiolytic-like effects observed with NPY and Y_1 receptor agonists in a variety of behavioural tests suggest that these compounds may have the potential to become an alternative to benzodiazepines for the treatment of anxiety-related disorders.

3.2 NPY and anxiety in human

Human studies have shown that acute, uncontrollable psychological stress significantly elevates plasma NPY levels, which were positively correlated with increased cortisol and norepinephrine concentrations. Enhanced NPY release was associated with less psychological dissociation suggesting that NPY exhibits anxiolytic activity during stress (Morgan et al. 2001). Increased NPY levels were detected in patients with chronic panic disorders who were drug-free for at least one week and had several panic attacks within one week before the procedure (Boulenger et al. 1996). Additionally, human studies in special operation soldiers under going extreme training showed that high NPY levels were associated with better performance (Morgan et al. 2000). Moreover, veteran patients with PTSD have been shown to have reduced plasma NPY levels as compared to veteran control subjects (Rasmusson et al. 2000).

3.3 NPY knockout and transgenic animals

Pharmacological studies consistently suggest that NPY is involved in the regulation of anxiety. However, from a behavioural perspective, pharmacological investigations can be complicated by the solubility of the compound used, its side effects and issues associated with handling and necessary restrain during the injection process (acute stress). On the other hand, the phenotypic changes observed in knockout animals as well as transgenic NPY animals are not as dramatic as might have been expected on the basis of pharmacological and morphological studies, possibly due to compensatory mechanisms. Furthermore, it is crucial to use a comprehensive behavioural phenotyping strategy when characterizing a genetic animal model including handling stress, circadian rhythms, locomotor activity, pain related phenotype, sedation and aggressivity in order to avoid false-positive, false-negative or fragmentary results.

Early behavioural studies of NPY-KO mice developed by two different groups reported inconsistent and confounding behavioural phenotypes. While Palmiter and collaborators reported increased anxiety-like behaviours in the elevated-plus maze and increased learning abilities in the passive avoidance task (Palmiter et al. 1998), Bannon et al. (2000) observed a wild-type (WT)-like performance for mice derived from the same line in both paradigms and an increase in anxiogenic-like behaviours in the open field test. Essentially, both studies were based solely on motor activity-dependent measures of anxiety rather than including a locomotion-independent parameter (i.e. ratio of motor activity in an aversive area or risk assessment behaviour) (Karl and Herzog 2007).

Most recently, Herzog and collaborators have developed new germline NPY-knockout mice which have been behaviourally characterized using a comprehensive multi-tiered phenotyping strategy (Karl et al. 2008). These newly developed NPY-KO mice consistently avoided aversive regions of the open field, light-dark box and elevated plus maze tests, as indicated by the time spent in these areas. Male NPY-deficient mice demonstrated a more potent and consistent anxiogenic phenotype than female NPY-KO mice, suggesting moderate sex-specific effects of NPY's deficiency. The potent anxious-like phenotype of NPY-deficient mice cannot simply be attributed to hypo-activity as the anxiogenic-like phenotype was confirmed by locomotion-independent parameters (i.e. ratio of distance travelled in aversive areas of the open field and light-dark box). In that context it is important to note that hypoactive NPY mutants did not show a complete absence of exploratory behaviours (reduced to 40–50% as compared to the wild type levels). Furthermore, stress-dependent measurements such as risk assessment behaviour (i.e. stretch–attend postures) and defecation score in the elevated plus maze also support an anxiogenic-like phenotype in NPY-deficient mice. The increased anxiety levels seen at baseline in NPY mutants are consistent with the extensive pharmacological data showing that NPY is an anxiolytic.

Transgenic animals overexpressing NPY have also been developed. Transgenic mice display behavioural signs of anxiety and hypertrophy of adrenal zona fasciculata cells, but no change in food intake was observed (Inui et al. 1998). The anxiety-like behavior of transgenic mice was reversed, at least in part, by the administration of CRF antagonists (alpha-helical CRF9-41) into the third ventricle. These results suggest that NPY plays a role in anxiety and behavioral responses to stress partly via the CRF neuronal system (Inui et al. 1998). Transgenic rat overexpressing NPY have also been developed by Michalkiewicz and his colleagues (Michalkiewicz and Michalkiewicz 2000) have been tested for anxiety-like behaviours. In this transgenic rat model, there is a central over-expression of prepro-NPY mRNA and NPY peptide in the hippocampus and hypothalamus, and decreased Y_1 binding sites within the hippocampus (Thorsell et al. 2000). These molecular and neurochemical events lead to altered anxiety profile and learning abilities in NPY-overexpressing rats. As observed in young NPY overexpressing rats, aged NPY-transgenic animals are resistant to acute physical restrain stress measured using the elevated-plus maze and demonstrate anxiolytic-like activity in the open field (Carvajal et al. 2004; Thorsell et al. 2000). These studies further support the role of NPY as a neuromodulator in the regulation of anxiety related behaviours throughout the lifespan.

3.4 Neuropeptide Y receptors

3.4.1 NPY Y_1 KO mice

Pharmacological studies demonstrated the role of NPY Y_1 receptor subtype in anxiety related behavioural tests. Accordingly, the lack of NPY Y_1 receptor signaling would predict an increase in anxiety-related behaviours. Several groups have generated NPY Y_1 receptor deficient mice, but they did not investigated in details the levels of anxiety in these animals until very recently. Early studies using NPY Y_1 KO mice showed increased ethanol consumption and reduced sensitivity to ethanol induced sedation (Thiele et al. 2002) which could be interpreted as secondary to high levels of anxiety. Additionally, the NPY Y_1 KO mice have an increase in locomotor activity and a strong increase in territorial but not spontaneous aggressive behaviours (Karl et al. 2004). However, and rather surprisingly, mice lacking the NPY Y_1 receptor subtype were found to be largely normal on tests of spontaneous anxiety-related behaviours (Karlsson et al. 2008). On the other hand, altered anxiety-like behaviours in NPY Y_1 KO mice appear to be highly dependent on the kind of task, time of testing within the circadian cycle, and stress exposure (Karl et al. 2006). Additionally, although NPY Y_1 KO mice do not show clear anxiogenic phenotype, they failed to respond to the anxiolytic-like effects of NPY (Karlsson et al. 2008).

3.4.2 NPY Y_2 KO mice

Studies using male mice deficient in the NPY Y_2 receptor subtype revealed that they have an anxiolytic-like phenotype in the elevated plus-maze and open field test with no changes in locomotor activity (Redrobe et al. 2003b). These findings were confirmed independently using the open field, elevated plus-maze, and light-dark compartment tests (Tschenett et al. 2003). However, an increase in locomotor activity was observed in the open field when mice were tested in light but not when tested in the dark (Tschenett et al. 2003). The anxiolytic-like profile of the Y2-deficient mice was confirmed in 2-yr-old Y_2 KO mice using the elevated plus-maze and open field test (Carvajal et al. 2006a). In agreement with the second study, an increase in locomotor activity in the open field was observed in NPY Y_2 KO mice compared to WT controls (Carvajal et al. 2006a). This is most likely because NPY Y_2 KO and WT control mice were tested in the open field with high light, rather than under low light conditions. More recently, another group has also shown that female NPY Y_2 KO mice spend more time in the open arms in the elevated plus maze test and enter more often in the central area in the open field test (Painsipp et al. 2008a), confirming the anxiolytic-like phenotype of the NPY Y_2 KO animals. However, they also demonstrated that the reduction of anxiety-related behaviour in Y_2 receptor KO animals were completely reversed by Escherichia coli lipopolysaccharide (LPS) (Painsipp et al. 2008a), with the anxiogenic-like effects most likely resulting from a reduction in locomotor activities after LPS.

3.4.3 NPY Y_4 KO mice

Male and female NPY Y_4 KO mice show very aggressive behaviour with increased incidents of fighting causing injuries between littermates (Sainsbury et al. 2002c). More recently, it has been reported that female NPY Y_4 KO display anxiolytic-like phenotypes similar to those seen with male NPY Y_2 KO mice as evaluated in the elevated plus maze and open field tests (Painsipp et al. 2008a; Painsipp et al. 2008b). Additionally, in the social interaction test, female NPY Y_4 KO mice had more contacts than wild type and NPY Y_2 KO mice (Painsipp et al. 2008a). These data suggest that in addition to Y_2 receptor antagonists, Y_4 receptor antagonists should be considered as an alternative in the treatment of mood and affective disorders. Interestingly, in contrast to NPY Y_2 KO mice (Redrobe et al. 2003a), NPY Y_4 KO mice did not show memory deficits (Painsipp et al. 2008b), suggesting that Y_4 receptor antagonists may be a more appropriate drug target for anxiety-related disorders as it may be less likely to induce memory deficits.

NPY Y_4, like Y_2, receptors are involved in the presynaptic inhibition of neurotransmitter release (Acuna-Goycolea et al. 2005), a mechanism that could explain why Y_4 receptor KO animals display similar alterations in emotional behaviours as Y_2 receptor KO mice. Additionally, the anxiolytic phenotype of NPY Y_4 KO mice is consistent with the anxiogenic phenotype observed in PP overexpressing mice (Ueno et al. 2007). Interestingly, icv injections of PP failed to alter anxiety-related behaviours (Asakawa et al. 1999), while chronic peripheral administration of PP reduced anxiety (Asakawa et al. 2003). It is also worth mentioning that both NPY Y_2 and Y_4 KO mice exhibit increased levels of circulating PP (Sainsbury et al. 2002a; Sainsbury et al. 2002c).

3.4.4 NPY Y_5 KO mice

Very little information is currently available regarding the mood and emotional status of NPY Y_5 KO mice. Central administration of neuropeptide Y (NPY) causes both anxiety and sedation as revealed by a decrease of locomotor activity in the open field (Heilig et al. 1989a; Heilig et al. 1989b; Heilig and Murison 1987; Redrobe et al. 2002a). Previous studies suggested that both effects are mediated via NPY Y_1 receptors, but as the $Y_1/Y_4/Y_5$ receptor agonist, [Leu^{31},Pro^{34}]PYY, causes sedation in the mouse open field test, it may suggest a role for Y_4 and Y_5 subtypes (Redrobe et al. 2002a). More recently, using more selective NPY agonists such as [D-His^{26}]NPY (Y_1), C2-NPY (Y_2), and [cPP1-7, NPY19-23, Ala^{31}, Aib^{32}, Gln^{34}]hPP (Y_5) in the elevated plus maze and open field tests, it was shown that anxiolytic-like effects of icv-administered NPY agonists in rats are mediated via both Y_1 and Y_5 receptors, whereas sedation mostly involves the Y_5 receptor (Sorensen et al. 2004). Further investigations based on more detailed behavioural phenotype of NPY Y_5 KO mice are required in order to clearly establish the role of the Y_5 receptor subtype in anxiety and sedation–related behaviours.

There are also unexpected differences between findings obtained in knockout and transgenic models, and pharmacological studies (Lin et al. 2004). Compensatory changes during development in knockout animals may explain the lack of phenotype observed in these animals. The use of knock-in strategies, which allows for the modification rather than the complete inactivation of receptor or ligand functions should be considered (Lin et al. 2004). Similarly, conditional KO models will also allow for the selective deletion of genes in a defined tissue or cell type of an adult animal, thereby avoiding compensatory mechanisms occurring during development.

4 Mechanims of action

In adult animals, exposure to stress was shown to alter NPY-related markers in many brain regions such as the amygdale, hippocampus, cortex, nucleus accumbens and caudate putamen (Table 3). For example, acute physical restrain which generates anxiety-like behaviour in a wide range of behavioural tests (Heilig 2004), also down-regulates the expression of NPY mRNA in the amygdala as well as the expression of NPY in this brain structure as well as in the frontal cortex (Thorsell et al. 1998). However, when rats are subjected to chronic stress, the anxiogenic-like behaviour was not observed and was accompanied by an up-regulation of pre-pro-NPY mRNA in the amygdala (Thorsell et al. 1999). The up-regulation of NPY mRNA following chronic stress suggests that NPY is involved in adaptive responses during exposure to stress.

The brain circuitry involved in mediating anxiety-related behavioural responses is complex and implicates not only the amygdala, but also the locus coeruleus, dorsal periaqueductal gray matter, septum, hippocampus and various hypothalamic nuclei (Kask et al. 2002).

The first anxiolytic drugs introduced on the market included benzodiazepines such as diazepam which act on GABA receptors. The co-localization of NPY and GABA in the amygdala (McDonald and Pearson 1989), hypothalamus (Horvath et al. 1997) and cerebral cortex (Aoki and Pickel 1989) and the existence of direct synaptic connections between GABA and NPY-ergic neurons in the amygdala (Oberto et al. 2001) and nucleus accumbens (Massari et al. 1988) as well as the co-localization of NPY Y_1 receptor subtype on GABA-ergic neurons in the amygdala (Oberto et al. 2001) all suggest that the anxiolytic properties of NPY could be mediated, at least partly, via GABA-ergic neurons. In support of this hypothesis, diazepam was shown to block the anxiogenic effects of BIBP3226, a Y_1 receptor antagonist (Kask et al. 1996). Moreover, alprozolam reduced anxiogenic-like behaviours induced by the Y_2 receptor agonist, C2-NPY in the social interaction test (Sajdyk et al. 2002). Additionally, it has been reported that the administration of diazepam and buspirone, an anxiolytic acting on the $5HT_{1A}$ receptor, in naïve rats resulted in a decrease in NPY-like ir in the amygdala and nucleus accumbens

Table 3. Effect of various stressors on NPY-related markers

Model of stress/fear	Results	Reference
Amygdala		
Restrain stress	50% increase NPY mRNA after 3 days	(Sweerts et al. 2001)
Conditioned fear produced in the passive avoidance test	33% increase in NPY-like ir after the test	(Krysiak et al. 2000)
Restrain stress	30 and 25 % decreased in NPY mRNA and NPY-like ir after 1 hr, respectively	(Thorsell et al. 1998)
Hypothalamus		
Restraint stress	81 and 40 % increased in NPY mRNA after 1 and 3 days, respectively (Arcuate nucleus)	(Sweerts et al. 2001)
Conditioned fear produced in the passive avoidance test	19% increase in NPY-like ir 6 hr after the test	(Krysiak et al. 2000)
Restraint stress	23% increase in NPY-like ir 10 hr after , no change in NPY mRNA	(Thorsell et al. 1998)
Cerebral cortex		
Conditioned fear produced in the passive avoidance test	21% increase in NPY-like ir 6 hr after the test	(Krysiak et al. 2000)
Restraint stress	35 and 45 % decrease in NPY mRNA 2 and 4 hr after, respectively. No change in NPY-like ir	(Thorsell et al. 1998)
Nucleus accumbens		
Conditioned fear produced in the passive avoidance test	22% increase in NPY-like ir 6 hr after the test	(Krysiak et al. 2000)
Hippocampus		
Restrain stress	26 % decrease in NPY mRNA after 10 days	(Sweerts et al. 2001)
Striatum		
Restraint stress	29 % increase in NPY mRNA 2 after. No change in NPY-like ir	(Thorsell et al. 1998)

(Krysiak et al. 1999). On the other hand, in rats subjected to conditioned fear, increases in NPY-like ir in the amygdala, nucleus accumbens and hypothalamus were blocked by diazepam and attenuated by buspirone (Krysiak et al. 2000). The effect of diazepam on brain NPY-like ir levels is also inhibited by the benzodiazepine receptor antagonist flumazenil (Krysiak et al. 2000). Interestingly chronic, but not acute, treatments with either diazepam or abecarnil produced significantly increases in the expression of the NPY Y_1 receptor subtype, while FG7142, an anxiogenic compound, decreased NPY Y_1 receptor expression (Oberto et al. 2000). Finally, the neurosteroid allopregnanolone demonstrates marked anxiolytic action by enhancing GABA-A receptor function and altered expression of the NPY Y_1 receptor in a similar fashion as diazepam and abecarnil (Ferrara et al. 2001).

Several lines of evidence suggest that the stimulation of group II and III metabotropic glutamate (mGlu) receptors produces anxiolytic-like effects in rodents (Smialowska et al. 2007; Wieronska et al. 2004; Wieronska et al. 2005). Interestingly, the anxiolytic effects of mGluR agonists are abolished by BIBO3304, a Y_1 receptor antagonist (Wieronska et al. 2005). More recently, it was reported that significant anxiolytic effects were induced by injection of group II and III mGlu agonists injected into the dentate gyrus and CA1 subfield of the hippocampus, respectively (Smialowska et al. 2007). NPY can also be anxiolytic following its injection into these structures. In the CA1 area, the effect of NPY is blocked by BIBO3304 (Y_1 antagonist), while BIIE0246 (Y_2 antagonist) was effective in the dentate gyrus (Smialowska et al. 2007). Similarly, BIBO3304 blocked the anxiolytic effect of group III mGlu agonists in the CA1 subfield while BIIE0246 was effective against Group II mGlu agonists injected in the dentate gyrus (Smialowska et al. 2007). Taken together, these data further demonstrate the complex neuronal circuitry implicated in anxiety-related behaviours and the possible role of the NPY Y_1 and Y_2 receptor subtypes in that regard.

CRF has been implicated in the coordination of behavioural and endocrine responses to stress (Koob and Heinrichs 1999). In contrast to NPY, central administration of CRF produced anxiogenic effects in several anxiety-related paradigms including the elevated plus maze, social interaction, conflict test and acoustic startle paradigm (Sajdyk et al. 2004). The anxiogenic effects of CRF in the social interaction, elevated plus maze and conflict test were all blocked by a pre-treatment with NPY (Britton et al. 2000; Kask et al. 2001). Additionally, deletion of the NPY Y_2 receptor induced a 70% reduction in CRF mRNA expression that might contribute to the anxiolytic-like phenotype observed in NPY Y_2 KO mice (Sainsbury et al. 2002b). Furthermore, thyroxine-treated adult animals displayed reduced anxiety and a decrease in the number of CRF-like ir neurons, but increased NPY-like ir neurons in the amygdala (Yilmazer-Hanke et al. 2004). All these data support previously proposed hypothesis that the two systems are closely inter-related and that NPY is important for dampening the effects of CRF under stressful conditions (Heilig et al. 1994).

5 The developmental theory of anxiety and NPY

There is increasing recognition that many psychiatric disorders including anxiety disorders could be, at least partly, of neurodevelopmental origin (Leonardo and Hen 2008). Data obtained in human and animal models point to a critical period during which neuronal circuits that mediate anxiety-like behaviours develop (Leonardo and Hen 2008). It has then been postulated that this highly plastic critical period is a time of heightened responsiveness that is particularly susceptible to adverse events (Leonardo and Hen 2008). Thus both anxiety trait and anxiety disorders are likely to be determined by early developmental processes or events that affect the way in which an individual brain is wired. Interestingly, while the mean age of onset of depression is 29, that of an anxiety disorder is 11 (Kessler et al. 2005). In fact, several studies in human indicated that exposure to early adverse life events can increase the vulnerability to both anxiety and depression into adulthood (Breslau et al. 1995; Ladd et al. 2000; Parker et al. 1995; Parker et al. 1999; Parker et al. 2000). The relationship between stressful events early in life and psychiatric disorders has been modeled in rats by subjecting them, for example, to early maternal deprivation. Maternal separation has been proposed as a potential experimental model for psychiatric conditions such as depression and/or anxiety disorders, and these animals exhibit increased anxiety "trait" in several paradigms (Caldji et al. 1998; Caldji et al. 2000; Huot et al. 2001; McIntosh et al. 1999). Additionally and in accordance with the potential role of NPY in anxiety, maternally-separated rats between postnatal days 2 -14 were shown to have lower NPY-like ir in the hippocampus, striatum, amygdala and cortex at three months of age (Husum et al. 2002; Husum and Mathe 2002; Jimenez-Vasquez et al. 2001; Park et al. 2005). Moreover, if lithium treatment was administered on days 50-83, changes in NPY-like ir induced by maternal deprivation were not observed (Husum and Mathe 2002). It has also been shown in this model that acupuncture treatment at acupoint Shenmen (HT7) reduces anxiety-like behaviours in adult rats and increased NPY expression in the amygdala (Park et al. 2005) and hippocampus (Lim et al. 2003) following maternal separation. These data demonstrate that early stressful events for a short period of time during development can have major and long lasting impacts on NPY contents in various brain regions as well as on anxiety-related "trait".

6 Developmental profile of NPY receptors

Considering the importance of brain development during the postnatal period, its role in psychiatric disorders and the evidence suggesting that NPY is involved in both anxious behaviours and brain development, we investigated the distribution of the NPY Y_1, Y_2, Y_4 and Y_5 receptor subtypes during brain development and maturation. Immunohistochemical studies have shown that NPY-immunoreactive materials are expressed in the embryonic rat brain as early as by day 13 (E13) with staining in perikarya being stronger prior to birth (Woodhams et al. 1985), suggesting that NPY may play a role during brain development. Furthermore, in situ hybridization studies have shown that the Y_1 receptor mRNA can be detected as early as by embryonic day 12 with levels of Y_1 mRNA transcripts increasing until birth with specific [^{125}I][Leu^{31},Pro^{34}]PYY binding sites having a similar pattern but delayed by 2 days (Tong et al. 1997). Additionally, RT-PCR studies have shown that the Y_1, Y_2 and Y_5 mRNAs are expressed very early in the brain, spinal cord and dorsal root ganglion of embryonic mouse (Naveilhan et al. 1998), and the Y_1 and Y_2 mRNAs in rat embryonic (E19) hippocampi (St Pierre et al. 1998). However, it is unclear if this is translated in the expression of their respective receptor protein since we failed for example, to detect specific [^{125}I]PYY3-36 binding in cultured primary E18-19 hippocampal neurons (St Pierre et al. 1998). We hence decided to investigate the respective distribution of the Y_1, Y_2, Y_4 and Y_5 receptor proteins in the brain from embryonic day 17 (E17) to postnatal day 90 (P90). Receptor autoradiography was performed as described in details elsewhere (Dumont et al. 1996; Dumont et al. 1998a; Dumont et al. 2000b; Dumont et al. 2000a; Dumont et al. 2005; Dumont and Quirion 2000). Briefly, on the day of the experiments, adjacent coronal sections were pre-incubated for 60 min at room temperature in a Krebs Ringer phosphate (KRP) buffer at pH 7.4 and then incubated in a fresh preparation of KRP buffer containing 0.1% bovine serum albumin (BSA), 0.05% bacitracin, 30 pM of either [^{125}I][Leu^{31},Pro^{34}]PYY and [^{125}I]GR231118 in the absence and presence of 100 nM BIBO3304 (Y_1 and Y_5-like receptors) (Dumont et al. 1998a; Dumont et al. 2000a; Dumont and Quirion 2000; Dumont and Quirion 2006), as well as [^{125}I]PYY3-36 (Y_2-like receptors) (Dumont et al. 2000b; Dumont et al. 2004), and [^{125}I]hPP (Y_4-like receptors) (Dumont et al. 2004; Dumont et al. 2005; Trinh et al. 1996). Following a 1 hr incubation for [^{125}I]GR231118 and 2.5 hr incubation for [^{125}I][Leu^{31},Pro^{34}]PYY, [^{125}I]PYY3-36 and [^{125}I]hPP, sections were washed four times, 1 min each in ice-cold KRP buffer, and then dipped in deionized water to remove salts and rapidly dried. Non-specific binding was determined in the presence of 1 µM [Leu^{31},Pro^{34}]PYY, 1 µM PYY3-36, 100 nM GR231118 and 100 nM hPP for [^{125}I][Leu^{31},Pro^{34}]PYY, [^{125}I]PYY3-36, [^{125}I]GR231118 and [^{125}I]hPP, respectively. Incubated sections were apposed against ^{3}H-Hyperfilms for 4 to 12 days alongside radioactive standards.

The NPY Y$_1$ receptor protein is detected at embryonic age (E17-E18) in various rat brain structures that also express the Y$_1$ receptor protein in the adult brain including the olfactory nuclei, cerebral cortex (especially in superficial layers), claustrum, thalamus, medial geniculate nucleus and various brainstem nuclei. The levels of specific [^{125}I]GR231118 and [^{125}I][Leu^{31},Pro^{34}]PYY/BIBO3304-sensitive binding sites increase gradually from E18 to reach adult levels by postnatal day P21 (Figs. 1 to 5). This pattern is seen for all brain structures including superficial layers of the cortex (Figs. 1-5), anterior olfactory nuclei, frontal (Fig. 1) and parietal (Fig. 2) cortices, striatum and lateral septum (Fig. 2), various thalamic and hypothalamic nuclei as well as the dorsal hippocampus and amygdala (Fig. 3), medial geniculate nucleus, substantia nigra (Fig. 4) and cerebellum, nucleus tractus solitarius and area postrema (Fig. 5) with gradual increases in specific binding for both Y$_1$ ligands from postnatal day P1 to adult levels by postnatal day P21.

The NPY Y$_2$ receptor protein is also detected at embryonic age (E17-E18) in rat brain structures that are distinct from those expressing the Y$_1$ receptor subtype. The most dramatic changes in distrubution and levels of expression occurring during ontogeny in the NPY family are seen with the Y$_2$ subtype. In cortical areas for example, while in the adult brain low levels of specific [^{125}I]PYY3-36 binding sites are detected, high amounts are seen in deep layers of the cortex at postnatal day P1 (Figs. 1-5). Moreover, levels of expression of Y$_2$ receptors increased to reach maximal values at P7 followed by marked decreases of specific [^{125}I]PYY3-36 binding thereafter to reach almost background levels by postnatal day P28 (Figs. 1-5). A similar pattern is also observed in the anterior olfactory nuclei (Fig. 1) as well as in the striatum and lateral septum (Fig. 2) and cerebellum (Fig. 5). However, in contrast to superficial cortical layers, in these brain regions significant amount of specific [^{125}I]PYY3-36 binding is still seen by postnatal day 21 and at levels similar to those seen in the adulthood. This developmental pattern is less pronounced in various thalamic and hypothalamic nuclei and hippocampus (Figs. 3-4). Interestingly, very high amounts of specific [^{125}I]PYY3-36 binding sites are already detected at the

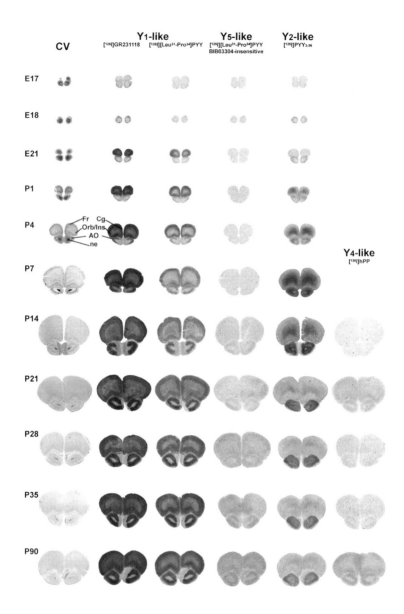

Fig 1. Photomicrographs of the autoradiographic distribution of [^{125}I]GR231118, [^{125}I][Leu^{31},Pro^{34}]PYY, [^{125}I][Leu^{31},Pro^{34}]PYY/BIBO3304-insensitive sites, [^{125}I]PYY3-36 and [^{125}I]hPP binding sites between embryonic day 17 (E17) and postnatal day 90 (P90) in at the level of the olfactory nuclei of the rat brain. AO: anterior olfactory nucleus; Cg: cingulate cortex; Fr: frontal cortex; Orb/Ins: orbital and insular cortex; ne: neuroepithelium.

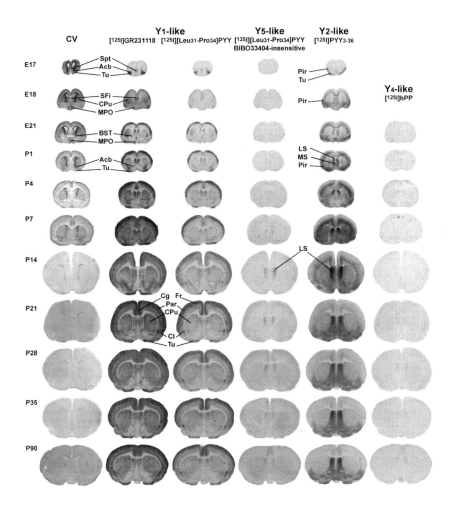

Fig. 2. Photomicrographs of the autoradiographic distribution of [^{125}I]GR231118, [^{125}I][Leu^{31},Pro^{34}]PYY, [^{125}I][Leu^{31},Pro^{34}]PYY/BIBO3304-insensitive sites, [^{125}I]PYY3-36 and [^{125}I]hPP binding sites between embryonic day 17 (E17) and postnatal day 90 (P90) at the level of the striatum of the rat brain. Acb: accumbens; BST: bed nucleus of the stria terminalis; Cg: cingulate cortex; Cl: claustrum; CPu: caudate putamen; Fr: frontal cortex; LS: lateral septum; MPO: medial preoptic nucleus; MS: medial septum; Par: parietal cortex; Pir: piriform cortex; SFi: septofimbrial nucleus; Spt: septum; Tu: olfactory tubercule.

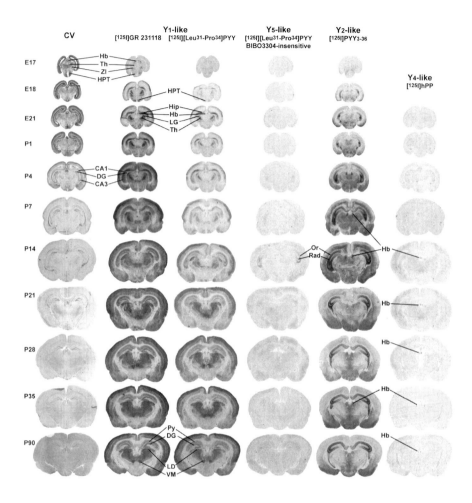

Fig. 3. Photomicrographs of the autoradiographic distribution of [^{125}I]GR231118, [^{125}I][Leu^{31},Pro^{34}]PYY, [^{125}I][Leu^{31},Pro^{34}]PYY/BIBO3304-insensitive sites, [^{125}I]PYY3-36 and [^{125}I]hPP binding sites between embryonic day 17 (E17) and postnatal day 90 (P90) at the level of the dorsal hippocampus of the rat brain. CA: fields of Hammon's horn; DG: dentate gyrus; Hb: habenula; Hip: hippocampus; HPT: hypothalamus; LD: laterodorsal thalamic nucleus; LG: lateral geniculate; Or: oriens layer of the hippocampus; Py: pyramidal cell layer of the hippocampus; Rad: stratum radiatum of the hippocampus; Th: thalamus; VM: ventromedial thalamic nucleus; ZI: zona incerta.

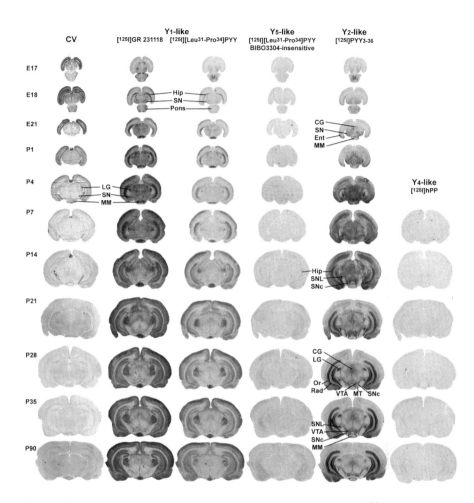

Fig. 4. Photomicrographs of the autoradiographic distribution of [^{125}I]GR231118, [^{125}I][Leu^{31},Pro^{34}]PYY, [^{125}I][Leu^{31},Pro^{34}]PYY/BIBO3304-insensitive sites, [^{125}I]PYY3-36 and [^{125}I]hPP binding sites between embryonic day 17 (E17) and postnatal day 90 (P90) at the level of the thalamus and substantia nigra of the rat brain. CG: central periaqueductal gray; Ent: entorhinal cortex; Hip: hippocampus; LG: lateral geniculate; MM: medial mammilary nucleus; MT: medial terminal nucleus of the accessory optic tract; Or: oriens layer of the hippocampus; Rad: stratum radiatum of the hippocampus; SNc: substantia nigra, compact part; SNL: substantia nigra, lateral part; VTA: ventral tegmental area.

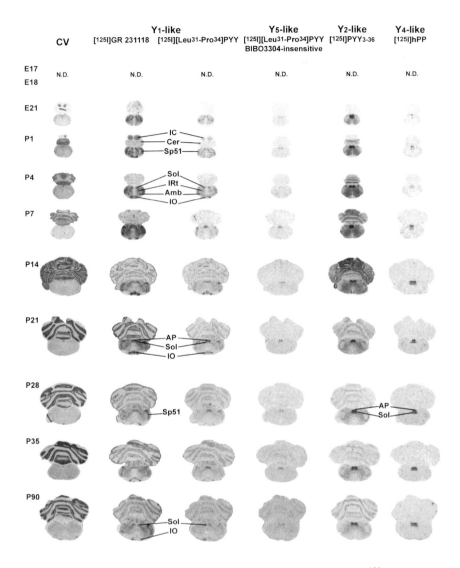

Fig. 5. Photomicrographs of the autoradiographic distribution of [^{125}I]GR231118, [^{125}I][Leu^{31},Pro^{34}]PYY, [^{125}I][Leu^{31},Pro^{34}]PYY/BIBO3304-insensitive sites, [^{125}I]PYY3-36 and [^{125}I]hPP binding sites between embryonic day 17 (E17) and postnatal day 90 (P90) at the level of the nucleus tractus solitarius of the rat brain. Amb: ambiguus nucleus; AP: area postrema; Cer: cerebellum; IC: inferior colliculus; IO: inferior olive; IRt: intermediate reticular zone; Sol: nucleus of the solitary tract; Sp5I: spinal trigeminal nucleus, interpolar part.

level of the nucleus tractus solitarius and area postrema as early as just before birth (E21) with levels remaining high after birth (Fig. 5).

In contrast to the Y_1 and Y_2 receptors, the Y_4 and Y_5 subtypes are detected only in very few brain regions (Figs. 1-5). The Y_4 subtype is seen only in the area postrema and nucleus tractus solitarius and is expressed as early as by embryonic day E21. Levels of specific $[^{125}I]hPP$ binding increased thereafter up to postnatal day P14 (Fig. 5). Early on, the Y_5 receptor subtype is detected in the lateral septum (Fig. 2), nucleus tractus solitarius and area postrema (Fig. 5). The developmental pattern of the Y_5 receptor subtype is similar to that of the Y_1 and Y_4 receptor subtypes. Significant amounts of specific $[^{125}I][Leu^{31},Pro^{34}]PYY/BIBO3304$-insensitive binding were particularly seen at postnatal day 1, reaching maximal levels by postnatal day P14-P21.

Considering that the critical period for the development of anxiety-related behaviours has been established to occur between P4 and P21 (Leonardo and Hen 2008), as well pharmacological data suggesting that NPY can decrease GABAergic transmission through the activation of Y_2 receptors (Kash and Winder 2006), while increasing it via the Y_1 subtype (see above), it will be of interest to investigate the role of NPY receptors in the maternal separation paradigm in order to study possible effects on the ontogenic profile of the NPY Y_1 and Y_2 receptor subtypes, and their effects on the development of anxiety "trait" in adulthood.

7 References

Acuna-Goycolea C, Tamamaki N, Yanagawa Y, Obata K, van den Pol AN (2005) Mechanisms of neuropeptide Y, peptide YY, and pancreatic polypeptide inhibition of identified green fluorescent protein-expressing GABA neurons in the hypothalamic neuroendocrine arcuate nucleus. J.Neurosci 25:7406-7419

Albers HE, Ferris CF (1984) Neuropeptide Y: role in light-dark cycle entrainment of hamster circadian rhythms. Neurosci.Lett. 50:163-168

Aoki C, Pickel VM (1989) Neuropeptide Y in the cerebral cortex and the caudate-putamen nuclei: ultrastructural basis for interactions with GABAergic and non-GABAergic neurons. J.Neurosci. 9:4333-4354

Asakawa A, Inui A, Ueno N, Fujimiya M, Fujino MA, Kasuga M (1999) Mouse pancreatic polypeptide modulates food intake, while not influencing anxiety in mice. Peptides 20:1445-1448

Asakawa A, Inui A, Yuzuriha H, Ueno N, Katsuura G, Fujimiya M, Fujino MA, Niijima A, Meguid MM, Kasuga M (2003) Characterization of the effects of pancreatic polypeptide in the regulation of energy balance. Gastroenterology 124:1325-1336

Bannon AW, Seda J, Carmouche M, Francis JM, Norman MH, Karbon B, McCaleb ML (2000) Behavioral characterization of neuropeptide Y knockout mice. Brain Res. 868:79-87

Belzung C, Griebel G (2001) Measuring normal and pathological anxiety-like behaviour in mice: a review. Behav.Brain Res. 125:141-149

Blomqvist AG, Herzog H (1997) Y-receptor subtypes--how many more? Trends Neurosci. 20:294-298

Boulenger JP, Jerabek I, Jolicoeur FB, Lavallee YJ, Leduc R, Cadieux A (1996) Elevated plasma levels of neuropeptide Y in patients with panic disorder. Am.J.Psychiatry 153:114-116

Breslau N, Schultz L, Peterson E (1995) Sex differences in depression: a role for preexisting anxiety. Psychiatry Res. 58:1-12

Britton KT, Southerland S, Van Uden E, Kirby D, Rivier J, Koob G (1997) Anxiolytic activity of NPY receptor agonists in the conflict test. Psychopharmacology (Berl) 132:6-13

Britton KT, Akwa Y, Spina MG, Koob GF (2000) Neuropeptide Y blocks anxiogenic-like behavioral action of corticotropin-releasing factor in an operant conflict test and elevated plus maze. Peptides 21:37-44

Broqua PP, Wettstein JJ, Rocher MM, Gauthier-Martin BB, Junien JJ (1995) Behavioral effects of neuropeptide Y receptor agonists in the elevated plus-maze and fear-potentiated startle procedures. Behav.Pharmacol. 6:215-222

Caldji C, Tannenbaum B, Sharma S, Francis D, Plotsky PM, Meaney MJ (1998) Maternal care during infancy regulates the development of neural systems mediating the expression of fearfulness in the rat. Proc.Natl.Acad.Sci.U.S A 95:5335-5340

Caldji C, Francis D, Sharma S, Plotsky PM, Meaney MJ (2000) The effects of early rearing environment on the development of GABAA and central benzodiazepine receptor levels and novelty-induced fearfulness in the rat. Neuropsychopharmacology 22:219-229

Carvajal CC, Vercauteren F, Dumont Y, Michalkiewicz M, Quirion R (2004) Aged neuropeptide Y transgenic rats are resistant to acute stress but maintain spatial and non-spatial learning. Behav.Brain Res. 153:471-480

Carvajal C, Dumont Y, Herzog H, Quirion R (2006a) Emotional behavior in aged neuropeptide Y (NPY) Y2 knockout mice. J.Mol.Neurosci 28:239-245

Carvajal C, Dumont Y, Quirion R (2006b) Neuropeptide Y: role in emotion and alcohol dependence. CNS Neurol.Disord.Drug Targets 5:181-195

Carvajal C, Dumont Y, Quirion R (2007) Neuropeptide Y. In: Fink G (ed) Encyclopedia of Stress, Second Edition, Volume 2. Academic Press, Oxford, UK, pp 895-903

Clark JT, Kalra PS, Kalra SP (1985) Neuropeptide Y stimulates feeding but inhibits sexual behavior in rats. Endocrinology 117:2435-2442

Colmers WF, Lukowiak K, Pittman QJ (1987) Presynaptic action of neuropeptide Y in area CA1 of the rat hippocampal slice. J.Physiol (Lond) 383:285-299

Dumont Y, Quirion R (2000) [125I]-GR231118: a high affinity radioligand to investigate neuropeptide Y Y1 and Y4 receptors. Br.J.Pharmacol. 129:37-46

Dumont Y, Quirion R (2006) An overview of neuropeptide Y: pharmacology to molecular biology and receptor localization. In: Zukowska Z, Feuerstein GZ (eds) NPY Family of Peptides in Neurobiology, Cardiovascular and Metabolism Disorders: from Genes to Therapeutics. Birkhauser Verlag, Berlin, Germany, pp 7-33

Dumont Y, Fournier A, St Pierre S, Quirion R (1996) Autoradiographic distribution of[125I][Leu31,Pro34]PYY and [125I]PYY3-36 binding sites in the rat brain evaluated with two newly developed Y1 and Y2 receptor radioligands. Synapse 22:139-158

Dumont Y, Fournier A, Quirion R (1998a) Expression and characterization of the neuropeptide Y Y5 receptor subtype in the rat brain. J.Neurosci. 18:5565-5574

Dumont Y, Jacques D, Bouchard P, Quirion R (1998b) Species differences in the expression and distribution of the neuropeptide Y Y1, Y2, Y4 and Y5 receptors in rodents, guinea pig and primates brains. J.Comp Neurol. 402:372-384

Dumont Y, Cadieux A, Doods H, Fournier A, Quirion R (2000a) Potent and selective tools to investigate neuropeptide Y receptors in the central and peripheral nervous systems: BIB03304 (Y1) and CGP71683A (Y5). Can.J.Physiol Pharmacol. 78:116-125

Dumont Y, Cadieux A, Doods H, Pheng LH, Abounader R, Hamel E, Jacques D, Regoli D, Quirion R (2000b) BIIE0246, a potent and highly selective nonpeptide neuropeptide Y Y2 receptor antagonist. Br.J.Pharmacol. 129:1075-1088

Dumont Y, Jacques D, St Pierre JA, Tong Y, Parker R, Herzog H, Quirion R (2000c) Neuropeptide Y, peptide YY and pancreatic polypeptide receptor proteins and mRNAs in mammalian brains. In: Quirion R, Bjorklund A, Hokfelt T (eds) Handbook of Chemical Neuroanatomy, Vol 16 Peptide Receptors, Part 1. Elsevier, London, UK, pp 375-475

Dumont Y, Chabot JG, Quirion R (2004) Receptor autoradiography as mean to explore the possible functional relevance of neuropeptides: Focus on new agonists and antagonists to study natriuretic peptides, neuropeptide Y and calcitonin gene-related peptides. Peptides 25:365-391

Dumont Y, Moyse E, Fournier A, Quirion R (2005) Evidence for the existence of an additional class of neuropeptide Y receptor sites in the rat brain. J.Pharmacol.Exp.Ther. 315:99-108

Edvinsson L, Ekblad E, Hakanson R, Wahlestedt C (1984) Neuropeptide Y potentiates the effect of various vasoconstrictor agents on rabbit blood vessels. Br.J.Pharmacol. 83:519-525

Ekman R, Wahlestedt C, Bottcher G, Sundler F, Hakanson R, Panula P (1986) Peptide YY-like immunoreactivity in the central nervous system of the rat. Regul.Pept. 16:157-168

Esteban J, Chover AJ, Sanchez PA, Mico JA, Gibert-Rahola J (1989) Central administration of neuropeptide Y induces hypothermia in mice. Possible interaction with central noradrenergic systems. Life Sci. 45:2395-2400

Ferrara G, Serra M, Zammaretti F, Pisu MG, Panzica GC, Biggio G, Eva C (2001) Increased expression of the neuropeptide Y receptor Y(1) gene in the medial amygdala of transgenic mice induced by long-term treatment with progesterone or allopregnanolone. J.Neurochem. 79:417-425

File SE, Lippa AS, Beer B, Lippa MT (2004) Animal tests of anxiety. Curr.Protoc.Neurosci Chapter 8:Unit

Flood JF, Hernandez EN, Morley JE (1987) Modulation of memory processing by neuropeptide Y. Brain Res. 421:280-290

Griebel G (1999) Is there a future for neuropeptide receptor ligands in the treatment of anxiety disorders? Pharmacol.Ther. 82:1-61

Harfstrand A (1986) Intraventricular administration of neuropeptide Y (NPY) induces hypotension, bradycardia and bradypnoea in the awake unrestrained male rat. Counteraction by NPY-induced feeding behaviour. Acta Physiol Scand. 128:121-123

Heilig M (1995) Antisense inhibition of neuropeptide Y (NPY)-Y1 receptor expression blocks the anxiolytic-like action of NPY in amygdala and paradoxically increases feeding. Regul.Pept. 59:201-205

Heilig M (2004) The NPY system in stress, anxiety and depression. Neuropeptides 38:213-224

Heilig M, Murison R (1987) Intracerebroventricular neuropeptide Y suppresses open field and home cage activity in the rat. Regul.Pept. 19:221-231

Heilig M, Soderpalm B, Engel JA, Widerlov E (1989a) Centrally administered neuropeptide Y (NPY) produces anxiolytic-like effects in animal anxiety models. Psychopharmacology (Berl) 98:524-529

Heilig M, Vecsei L, Widerlov E (1989b) Opposite effects of centrally administered neuropeptide Y (NPY) on locomotor activity of spontaneously hypertensive (SH) and normal rats. Acta Physiol Scand. 137:243-248

Heilig M, McLeod S, Koob GK, Britton KT (1992) Anxiolytic-like effect of neuropeptide Y (NPY), but not other peptides in an operant conflict test. Regul.Pept. 41:61-69

Heilig M, McLeod S, Brot M, Heinrichs SC, Menzaghi F, Koob GF, Britton KT (1993) Anxiolytic-like action of neuropeptide Y: mediation by Y1 receptors in amygdala, and dissociation from food intake effects. Neuropsychopharmacology 8:357-363

Heilig M, Koob GF, Ekman R, Britton KT (1994) Corticotropin-releasing factor and neuropeptide Y: role in emotional integration. Trends Neurosci. 17:80-85

Horvath TL, Bechmann I, Naftolin F, Kalra SP, Leranth C (1997) Heterogeneity in the neuropeptide Y-containing neurons of the rat arcuate nucleus: GABAergic and non-GABAergic subpopulations. Brain Res. 756:283-286

Huot RL, Thrivikraman KV, Meaney MJ, Plotsky PM (2001) Development of adult ethanol preference and anxiety as a consequence of neonatal maternal separation in Long Evans rats and reversal with antidepressant treatment. Psychopharmacology (Berl) 158:366-373

Husum H, Mathe AA (2002) Early life stress changes concentrations of neuropeptide Y and corticotropin-releasing hormone in adult rat brain. Lithium treatment modifies these changes. Neuropsychopharmacology 27:756-764

Husum H, Termeer E, Mathe AA, Bolwig TG, Ellenbroek BA (2002) Early maternal deprivation alters hippocampal levels of neuropeptide Y and calcitonin-gene related peptide in adult rats. Neuropharmacology 42:798-806

Inui A (2000) Transgenic approach to the study of body weight regulation. Pharmacol.Rev. 52:35-61

Inui A, Okita M, Nakajima M, Momose K, Ueno N, Teranishi A, Miura M, Hirosue Y, Sano K, Sato M, Watanabe M, Sakai T, Watanabe T, Ishida K, Silver J, Baba S, Kasuga M (1998) Anxiety-like behavior in transgenic mice with brain expression of neuropeptide Y. Proc.Assoc.Am.Physicians 110:171-182

Jimenez-Vasquez PA, Mathe AA, Thomas JD, Riley EP, Ehlers CL (2001) Early maternal separation alters neuropeptide Y concentrations in selected brain regions in adult rats. Brain Res.Dev.Brain Res. 131:149-152

Kalra SP, Crowley WR (1984) Differential effects of pancreatic polypeptide on luteinizing hormone release in female rats. Neuroendocrinology 38:511-513

Kalra SP, Kalra PS (2006) Neuropeptide Y: A conductor of the appetite-regulating orchestra in the hypothalamus. In: Kastin AJ (ed) Handbook of Biologically Active Peptides. Acadenic Press, San Diego, USA, pp 889-894

Karl T, Herzog H (2007) Behavioral profiling of NPY in aggression and neuropsychiatric diseases. Peptides 28:326-333

Karl T, Lin S, Schwarzer C, Sainsbury A, Couzens M, Wittmann W, Boey D, von Horsten S, Herzog H (2004) Y1 receptors regulate aggressive behavior by modulating serotonin pathways. Proc.Natl.Acad.Sci.U.S.A 101:12742-12747

Karl T, Burne TH, Herzog H (2006) Effect of Y1 receptor deficiency on motor activity, exploration, and anxiety. Behav.Brain Res. 167:87-93

Karl T, Duffy L, Herzog H (2008) Behavioural profile of a new mouse model for NPY deficiency. Eur.J.Neurosci 28:173-180

Karlsson RM, Holmes A, Heilig M, Crawley JN (2005) Anxiolytic-like actions of centrally-administered neuropeptide Y, but not galanin, in C57BL/6J mice. Pharmacol.Biochem.Behav. 80:427-436

Karlsson RM, Choe JS, Cameron HA, Thorsell A, Crawley JN, Holmes A, Heilig M (2008) The neuropeptide Y Y1 receptor subtype is necessary for the anxiolytic-like effects of neuropeptide Y, but not the antidepressant-like effects of fluoxetine, in mice. Psychopharmacology (Berl) 195:547-557

Kash TL, Winder DG (2006) Neuropeptide Y and corticotropin-releasing factor bi-directionally modulate inhibitory synaptic transmission in the bed nucleus of the stria terminalis. Neuropharmacology 51:1013-1022

Kask A, Rago L, Harro J (1996) Anxiogenic-like effect of the neuropeptide Y Y1 receptor antagonist BIBP3226: antagonism with diazepam. Eur.J.Pharmacol. 317:R3-R4

Kask A, Nguyen HP, Pabst R, von Horsten S (2001) Neuropeptide Y Y1 receptor-mediated anxiolysis in the dorsocaudal lateral septum: functional antagonism of corticotropin-releasing hormone-induced anxiety. Neuroscience 104:799-806

Kask A, Harro J, von Horsten S, Redrobe JP, Dumont Y, Quirion R (2002) The neurocircuitry and receptor subtypes mediating anxiolytic-like effects of neuropeptide Y. Neurosci.Biobehav.Rev. 26:259-283

Kessler RC, Berglund P, Demler O, Jin R, Merikangas KR, Walters EE (2005) Lifetime prevalence and age-of-onset distributions of DSM-IV disorders in the National Comorbidity Survey Replication. Arch.Gen.Psychiatry 62:593-602

Klapstein GJ, Colmers WF (1997) Neuropeptide Y suppresses epileptiform activity in rat hippocampus in vitro. J.Neurophysiol. 78:1651-1661

Koob GF, Heinrichs SC (1999) A role for corticotropin releasing factor and urocortin in behavioral responses to stressors. Brain Res. 848:141-152

Krysiak R, Obuchowicz E, Herman ZS (1999) Diazepam and buspirone alter neuropeptide Y-like immunoreactivity in rat brain. Neuropeptides 33:542-549

Krysiak R, Obuchowicz E, Herman ZS (2000) Conditioned fear-induced changes in neuropeptide Y-like immunoreactivity in rats: the effect of diazepam and buspirone. Neuropeptides 34:148-157

Ladd CO, Huot RL, Thrivikraman KV, Nemeroff CB, Meaney MJ, Plotsky PM (2000) Long-term behavioral and neuroendocrine adaptations to adverse early experience. Prog.Brain Res. 122:81-103

Larhammar D (1996) Evolution of neuropeptide Y, peptide YY and pancreatic polypeptide. Regul.Pept. 62:1-11

Leonardo ED, Hen R (2008) Anxiety as a developmental disorder. Neuropsychopharmacology 33:134-140

Lim S, Ryu YH, Kim ST, Hong MS, Park HJ (2003) Acupuncture increases neuropeptide Y expression in hippocampus of maternally-separated rats. Neurosci.Lett. 343:49-52

Lin S, Boey D, Herzog H (2004) NPY and Y receptors: lessons from transgenic and knockout models. Neuropeptides 38:189-200

Massari VJ, Chan J, Chronwall BM, O'Donohue TL, Oertel WH, Pickel VM (1988) Neuropeptide Y in the rat nucleus accumbens: ultrastructural localization in aspiny neurons receiving synaptic input from GABAergic terminals. J.Neurosci.Res. 19:171-186

Mathew SJ, Price RB, Charney DS (2008) Recent advances in the neurobiology of anxiety disorders: implications for novel therapeutics. Am.J.Med.Genet.C.Semin.Med.Genet. 148:89-98

McDonald AJ, Pearson JC (1989) Coexistence of GABA and peptide immunoreactivity in non-pyramidal neurons of the basolateral amygdala. Neurosci.Lett. 100:53-58

McEwen BS (2000) The neurobiology of stress: from serendipity to clinical relevance. Brain Res. 886:172-189

McIntosh J, Anisman H, Merali Z (1999) Short- and long-periods of neonatal maternal separation differentially affect anxiety and feeding in adult rats: gender-dependent effects. Brain Res.Dev.Brain Res. 113:97-106

Michalkiewicz M, Michalkiewicz T (2000) Developing transgenic neuropeptide Y rats. Methods Mol.Biol. 153:73-89:73-89

Michel MC, Beck-Sickinger A, Cox H, Doods HN, Herzog H, Larhammar D, Quirion R, Schwartz T, Westfall T (1998) XVI. International Union of Pharmacology recommendations for the nomenclature of neuropeptide Y, peptide YY, and pancreatic polypeptide receptors. Pharmacol.Rev. 50:143-150

Millan MJ (2003) The neurobiology and control of anxious states. Prog.Neurobiol. 70:83-244

Morgan CA, Wang S, Southwick SM, Rasmusson A, Hazlett G, Hauger RL, Charney DS (2000) Plasma neuropeptide-Y concentrations in humans exposed to military survival training. Biol.Psychiatry 47:902-909

Morgan CA, Wang S, Rasmusson A, Hazlett G, Anderson G, Charney DS (2001) Relationship among plasma cortisol, catecholamines, neuropeptide Y, and human performance during exposure to uncontrollable stress. Psychosom.Med. 63:412-422

Nakajima M, Inui A, Asakawa A, Momose K, Ueno N, Teranishi A, Baba S, Kasuga M (1998) Neuropeptide Y produces anxiety via Y2-type receptors. Peptides 19:359-363

Naveilhan P, Neveu I, Arenas E, Ernfors P (1998) Complementary and overlapping expression of Y1, Y2 and Y5 receptors in the developing and adult mouse nervous system. Neuroscience 87:289-302

Naveilhan P, Canals JM, Valjakka A, Vartiainen J, Arenas E, Ernfors P (2001) Neuropeptide Y alters sedation through a hypothalamic Y1-mediated mechanism. Eur.J.Neurosci. 13:2241-2246

Nemeroff CB (2003) Anxiolytics: past, present, and future agents. J.Clin.Psychiatry 64 Suppl 3:3-6

Oberto A, Panzica G, Altruda F, Eva C (2000) Chronic modulation of the GABA(A) receptor complex regulates Y1 receptor gene expression in the medial amygdala of transgenic mice. Neuropharmacology 39:227-234

Oberto A, Panzica GC, Altruda F, Eva C (2001) GABAergic and NPY-Y(1) network in the medial amygdala: a neuroanatomical basis for their functional interaction. Neuropharmacology 41:639-642

Painsipp E, Herzog H, Holzer P (2008a) Implication of neuropeptide-Y Y2 receptors in the effects of immune stress on emotional, locomotor and social behavior of mice. Neuropharmacology 55:117-126

Painsipp E, Wultsch T, Edelsbrunner ME, Tasan RO, Singewald N, Herzog H, Holzer P (2008b) Reduced anxiety-like and depression-related behavior in neuropeptide Y Y4 receptor knockout mice. Genes Brain Behav. 7:532-542

Palmiter RD, Erickson JC, Hollopeter G, Baraban SC, Schwartz MW (1998) Life without neuropeptide Y. Recent Prog.Horm.Res. 53:163-99:163-199

Park HJ, Chae Y, Jang J, Shim I, Lee H, Lim S (2005) The effect of acupuncture on anxiety and neuropeptide Y expression in the basolateral amygdala of maternally separated rats. Neurosci Lett. 377:179-184

Parker G, Hadzi-Pavlovic D, Greenwald S, Weissman M (1995) Low parental care as a risk factor to lifetime depression in a community sample. J.Affect.Disord. 33:173-180

Parker G, Wilhelm K, Mitchell P, Austin MP, Roussos J, Gladstone G (1999) The influence of anxiety as a risk to early onset major depression. J.Affect.Disord. 52:11-17

Parker G, Gladstone G, Mitchell P, Wilhelm K, Roy K (2000) Do early adverse experiences establish a cognitive vulnerability to depression on exposure to mirroring life events in adulthood? J.Affect.Disord. 57:209-215

Pich EM, Agnati LF, Zini I, Marrama P, Carani C (1993) Neuropeptide Y produces anxiolytic effects in spontaneously hypertensive rats. Peptides 14:909-912

Rasmusson AM, Hauger RL, Morgan CA, Bremner JD, Charney DS, Southwick SM (2000) Low baseline and yohimbine-stimulated plasma neuropeptide Y (NPY) levels in combat-related PTSD. Biol.Psychiatry 47:526-539

Redrobe JP, Dumont Y, Fournier A, Quirion R (2002a) The Neuropeptide Y (NPY) Y1 Receptor Subtype Mediates NPY-induced Antidepressant-like Activity in the Mouse Forced Swimming Test. Neuropsychopharmacology 26:615-624

Redrobe JP, Dumont Y, Quirion R (2002b) Neuropeptide Y (NPY) and depression: From animal studies to the human condition. Life Sci. 71:2921-2937

Redrobe JP, Dumont Y, Herzog H, Quirion R (2003a) Characterization of neuropeptide Y, Y2 receptor knockout mice in two animal models of learning and memory processing. J.Mol.Neurosci. 22:159-166

Redrobe JP, Dumont Y, Herzog H, Quirion R (2003b) Neuropeptide Y (NPY) Y(2) receptors mediate behaviour in two animal models of anxiety: evidence from Y(2) receptor knockout mice. Behav.Brain Res. 141:251-255

Sainsbury A, Schwarzer C, Couzens M, Fetissov S, Furtinger S, Jenkins A, Cox HM, Sperk G, Hokfelt T, Herzog H (2002a) Important role of hypothalamic Y2 receptors in body weight regulation revealed in conditional knockout mice. Proc.Natl.Acad.Sci.U.S.A 99:8938-8943

Sainsbury A, Schwarzer C, Couzens M, Herzog H (2002b) Y2 receptor deletion attenuates the type 2 diabetic syndrome of ob/ob mice. Diabetes 51:3420-3427

Sainsbury A, Schwarzer C, Couzens M, Jenkins A, Oakes SR, Ormandy CJ, Herzog H (2002c) Y4 receptor knockout rescues fertility in ob/ob mice. Genes Dev. 16:1077-1088

Sajdyk TJ, Vandergriff MG, Gehlert DR (1999) Amygdalar neuropeptide Y Y1 receptors mediate the anxiolytic-like actions of neuropeptide Y in the social interaction test. Eur.J.Pharmacol. 368:143-147

Sajdyk TJ, Schober DA, Smiley DL, Gehlert DR (2002) Neuropeptide Y-Y(2) receptors mediate anxiety in the amygdala. Pharmacol.Biochem.Behav. 71:419-423

Sajdyk TJ, Shekhar A, Gehlert DR (2004) Interactions between NPY and CRF in the amygdala to regulate emotionality. Neuropeptides 38:225-234

Smialowska M, Wieronska JM, Domin H, Zieba B (2007) The effect of intrahippocampal injection of group II and III metobotropic glutamate receptor agonists on anxiety; the role of neuropeptide Y. Neuropsychopharmacology 32:1242-1250

Sorensen G, Lindberg C, Wortwein G, Bolwig TG, Woldbye DP (2004) Differential roles for neuropeptide Y Y1 and Y5 receptors in anxiety and sedation. J.Neurosci.Res. 77:723-729

Southwick SM, Vythilingam M, Charney DS (2005) The psychobiology of depression and resilience to stress: implications for prevention and treatment. Annu.Rev.Clin.Psychol. 1:255-291

St Pierre JA, Dumont Y, Nouel D, Herzog H, Hamel E, Quirion R (1998) Preferential expression of the neuropeptide Y Y1 over the Y2 receptor subtype in cultured hippocampal neurons and cloning of the rat Y2 receptor. Br.J.Pharmacol. 123:183-194

Stanley BG, Leibowitz SF (1984) Neuropeptide Y: stimulation of feeding and drinking by injection into the paraventricular nucleus. Life Sci. 35:2635-2642

Sweerts BW, Jarrott B, Lawrence AJ (2001) The effect of acute and chronic restraint on the central expression of prepro-neuropeptide Y mRNA in normotensive and hypertensive rats. J.Neuroendocrinol. 13:608-617

Tatemoto K (1982) Neuropeptide Y: complete amino acid sequence of the brain peptide. Proc.Natl.Acad.Sci.U.S.A 79:5485-5489

Thiele TE, Marsh DJ, Marie L, Bernstein IL, Palmiter RD (1998) Ethanol consumption and resistance are inversely related to neuropeptide Y levels. Nature 396:366-369

Thiele TE, Koh MT, Pedrazzini T (2002) Voluntary alcohol consumption is controlled via the neuropeptide Y Y1 receptor. J.Neurosci. 22:RC208

Thorsell A, Carlsson K, Ekman R, Heilig M (1999) Behavioral and endocrine adaptation, and up-regulation of NPY expression in rat amygdala following repeated restraint stress. Neuroreport 10:3003-3007

Thorsell A, Svensson P, Wiklund L, Sommer W, Ekman R, Heilig M (1998) Suppressed neuropeptide Y (NPY) mRNA in rat amygdala following restraint stress. Regul.Pept. 75-76:247-254

Thorsell A, Michalkiewicz M, Dumont Y, Quirion R, Caberlotto L, Rimondini R, Mathe AA, Heilig M (2000) Behavioral insensitivity to restraint stress, absent fear suppression of behavior and impaired spatial learning in transgenic rats with hippocampal neuropeptide Y overexpression. Proc.Natl.Acad.Sci.U.S.A 97:12852-12857

Tong Y, Dumont Y, Shen SH, Quirion R (1997) Comparative developmental profile of the neuropeptide Y Y1 receptor gene and protein in the rat brain. Mol.Brain Res. 48:323-332

Trinh T, Dumont Y, Quirion R (1996) High levels of specific neuropeptide Y/pancreatic polypeptide receptors in the rat hypothalamus and brainstem. Eur.J.Pharmacol. 318:R1-R3

Tsagarakis S, Rees LH, Besser GM, Grossman A (1989) Neuropeptide-Y stimulates CRF-41 release from rat hypothalami in vitro. Brain Res. 502:167-170

Tschenett A, Singewald N, Carli M, Balducci C, Salchner P, Vezzani A, Herzog H, Sperk G (2003) Reduced anxiety and improved stress coping ability in mice lacking NPY-Y2 receptors. Eur.J.Neurosci. 18:143-148

Ueno N, Asakawa A, Satoh Y, Inui A (2007) Increased circulating cholecystokinin contributes to anorexia and anxiety behavior in mice overexpressing pancreatic polypeptide. Regul.Pept. 141:8-11

Vezzani A, Sperk G, Colmers WF (1999) Neuropeptide Y: emerging evidence for a functional role in seizure modulation. Trends Neurosci. 22:25-30

Wahlestedt C, Hakanson R (1986) Effects of neuropeptide Y (NPY) at the sympathetic neuroeffector junction. Can pre- and postjunctional receptors be distinguished? Med.Biol. 64:85-88

Wahlestedt C, Pich EM, Koob GF, Yee F, Heilig M (1993) Modulation of anxiety and neuropeptide Y-Y1 receptors by antisense oligodeoxynucleotides. Science 259:528-531

Wang JZ, Lundeberg T, Yu L (2000) Antinociceptive effects induced by intraperiaqueductal grey administration of neuropeptide Y in rats. Brain Res. 859:361-363

Wieronska JM, Smialowska M, Branski P, Gasparini F, Klodzinska A, Szewczyk B, Palucha A, Chojnacka-Wojcik E, Pilc A (2004) In the amygdala anxiolytic action of mGlu5 receptors antagonist MPEP involves neuropeptide Y but not GABAA signaling. Neuropsychopharmacology 29:514-521

Wieronska JM, Szewczyk B, Palucha A, Branski P, Zieba B, Smialowska M (2005) Anxiolytic action of group II and III metabotropic glutamate receptors agonists involves neuropeptide Y in the amygdala. Pharmacol.Rep. 57:734-743

Woodhams PL, Allen YS, McGovern J, Allen JM, Bloom SR, Balazs R, Polak JM (1985) Immunohistochemical analysis of the early ontogeny of the neuropeptide Y system in rat brain. Neuroscience 15:173-202

Yilmazer-Hanke DM, Hantsch M, Hanke J, Schulz C, Faber-Zuschratter H, Schwegler H (2004) Neonatal thyroxine treatment: changes in the number of corticotropin-releasing-factor (CRF) and neuropeptide Y (NPY) containing neurons and density of tyrosine hydroxylase positive fibers (TH) in the amygdala correlate with anxiety-related behavior of wistar rats. Neuroscience 124:283-297

The search for a fetal origin for autism: evidence of aberrant brain development in a rat model of autism produced by prenatal exposure to valproate

Tetsuo Ogawa, Makiko Kuwagata, and Seiji Shioda

Department of Anatomy 1, Showa University, School of Medicine, 1-5-8 Hatanodai, Shinagawa-ku, Tokyo 142-8555, Japan

Summary. A variety of animal models for autism have been used to investigate autism, including models based on genetic manipulation (knockout) of candidate genes, and surgical lesions to specific brain regions. Most of these models have focused on the study of abnormalities observed in adult animals. We considered that the study of abnormalities at a fetal level might provide information concerning mechanisms underlying early developmental alterations that give rise to autism. For example, prenatal exposure to chemicals such as Valproate (VPA) has been clinically associated with an increased risk of autism in humans. Exposing pregnant rats to VPA has been reported to induce several behavioral and neurochemical anomalies associated with autism in offspring. Here, we have focused on developmental changes in fetal rat brains shortly after VPA exposure. We treated pregnant Sprague Dawley rats with VPA orally on gestation day 9 or 11, and observed different brain regions at embryonic day 16. VPA treatment on either day impaired development of the cortical plate in the cerebral cortex. We also detected an abnormal formation of nerve tracts and impaired migration and distribution of aminergic neurons in the hindbrain. These results suggest that the VPA-induced animal model of autism can reproduce, at least in part, some anatomopathological findings reported in idiopathic autism, and that such changes are already apparent in the fetal brain.

Key words. Autism, Valproate, Catecholamine, 5-HT, Fetal brain

1 Introduction

Autism is a neurodevelopmental disorder characterized by impaired social interaction, verbal and nonverbal communication, and restricted, repetitive, and stereotyped patterns of behavior, interests, and activities. Despite significant efforts to elucidate the pathophysiology and etiology of autistic disorders, their causes remain unknown. Epidemiological studies have demonstrated that some prenatal factors can increase the risk of autism. For example, maternal rubella infection (Chess, 1971), alcohol consumption (Nanson, 1992), thalidomide medication (Stromland et al., 1994), anticonvulsant medication (Moore et al., 2000), and misoprostol medication (Bandim et al., 2003), have been associated with an increased risk of autism in offspring (Reviewed by Arndt et al. 2005). Rasalam et al.(2005) investigated clinical features and the frequency of autism or Asperger syndrome in children exposed to anticonvulsant medication in utero. They reported that VPA was the drug most commonly associated with autism, five of 56 (8.9%) children in their study who had been exposed to sodium valproate had either autistic disorder or Asperger syndrome (Rasalam et al.2005). These epidemiological studies and other case reports are useful to investigate the timing of autism's origins. Timing of the impact which increases the risk can be obtained by interviewing mothers, or deduced from accompanying somatic defects in affected children. Children who have suffered prenatal exposure to VPA often exhibit dysmorphic features (e.g., neural tube defects, craniofacial abnormalities, abnormally shaped or posteriorly rotated ears, genital abnormalities, and limb defects) which are indicative of injury around the time of neural tube closure (Kozma 2001, Arndt et al. 2005).

Following these reports in humans, several studies have reported using an animal model of autism, obtained by exposing pregnant rats to VPA. This treatment has been reported to reproduce histological abnormalities in the brainstem nuclei and the cerebellum resembling those seen in human autistic cases (Rodier et al. 1997, Ingram et al. 2000). In addition, in utero exposure to VPA in rats has recently been demonstrated to induce behavioral alterations in offspring consistent with, or similar to, behavioral alterations reported in autistic children (Schneider and Przewlocki 2005, Stanton et al. 2007, Schneider et al. 2008, Nakasato et al. 2008). These studies administered VPA on gestation day (GD) 11-12, which corresponds to the period shortly after neural tube closure. Since "hyperserotonemia", that is an increase in blood levels of serotonin (5-HT), is typically exhibited by autistic children, some researchers have focused on the 5-HT nervous system in rats, and reported increased 5-HT in the brain and blood of offspring in response to exposure to VPA on GD 9 (Narita et al. 2002, Tsujino et al. 2007). All of above studies investigated offspring following prenatal VPA exposure. In considering the fetal origins of autistic spectrum disorders, it is both important and interesting to examine aspects of fetal brain development in the animal model of autism.

2 Methods

Pregnant Sprague-Dawley (Crl:CD, SD) rats were purchased on GD 3 or GD 4 from the Japan Charles River Laboratory (Atsugi, Japan). The rats were housed under conditions of controlled temperature and relative humidity, with a 12-12h light-dark cycle. Sodium valproate (VPA; Sigma, St. Louis, MO) was dissolved in saline immediately prior to use. VPA (800 mg/kg) was administered orally via gavage to pregnant rats on GD 9 (VPA9) or GD 11 (VPA11). As a vehicle control, saline (5 mL/kg) was administered. The dams were sacrificed on GD16. Preparation of fetal brains was followed as in our previous report (Ogawa, et al., 2005). Briefly, the fetal brains were fixed in 4 % paraformaldehyde in 0.1 M phosphate buffer. The brains were embedded in 10 % gelatin and coronal sections were cut with a vibratome at a thickness of 45 µm. For histopathological examinations, the serial sections in each group were stained with cresyl violet. In addition, serotonin (5-HT; polyclonal 5-HT antibody, 1:8000 dilution; ImmunoStar, WI), tyrosine hydroxylase (TH; polyclonal TH antibody, 1:1000 dilution; Pel-Freez, NA) and/or neuronal Class III beta-tubulin (monoclonal TuJ1 antibody, 1:2000 dilution; COVANCE, CA) immunohistochemistry was carried out following routine processes with the ABC method and visualization of the antigen using diaminobenzidine as a substrate.

3 Results

Images of sections showing the cerebral cortex of control and VPA-treated fetal brains at E 16 are given in Fig.1. In the control group, the structure of the cortical plate (CP) at which immature neurons accumulate after leaving the neuroepithelium layer can be clearly observed (Fig.1 A, arrow). However, the structure of the CP was not as evident in the brain sections of animals exposed to VPA at E 9 or E 11. This result suggests that prenatal exposure to VPA induced cortical dysgenesis in thses animals. TuJ1 immunohistochemistry highlighted this abnormality as an irregular distribution of immunoreactivities around the CP (data not shown). In the VPA11 group, an abnormally developed nerve tract, which was seen to have an irregular round structure in cresyl violet-stained sections, and was immunoreactive for TuJ1, could be identified in the hindbrain. This abnormal structure was not seen in sections from control and VPA9 groups (Fig.2 A,B,E,F). Further immunohistochemical observations revealed tyrosine hydroxylase- (TH-) immunoreactive neurons in the abnormally-developed nerve tract (Fig.2 G), and 5-HT-positive neurons around this structure (Fig.2 H), indicating that prenatal exposure to VPA caused an atypical migration of catecholaminergic neurons and an abnormal distribution of 5-HT neurons. These abnormalities were observed only in the VPA11 group, and in nearly 90% of animals in this group.

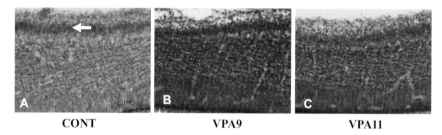

Fig.1 Cerebral cortex at E 16 after VPA exposure at E 9 or E 11. Fetal brain exposed to saline (CONT) in (A), to VPA at E 9 (VPA9) in (B) and to VPA at E 11 (VPA11) in (C). Arrow shows cortical plate. The structure of the cortical plate is less well-defined after VPA exposure at both E9 and E11.

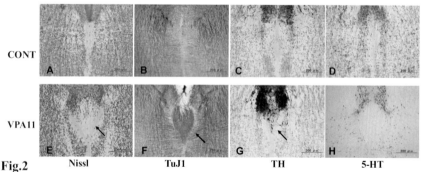

Fig.2 Hindbrain at E 16 after VPA exposure at E 9 or E 11. Fetal brain exposed to saline (CONT) in (A), (B), (C) and (D), and to VPA at E 11 (VPA11) in (E), (F), (G) and (H). Fetal brainsections stained with cresyl violet in (A) and (E), and stained immunohistochemically for TuJ1 in (B) and (F), for TH in (C) and (G), and for 5-HT in (D) and (H).

4 Discussion

Exposure of the fetal rat to VPA on GD 9 and 11 affected development of the cortical plate in the cerebral cortex, suggesting that VPA inhibited proliferation of the neural stem cells and/or migration of the immature neurons in the cerebral cortex. This finding is consistent with a clinicopathologic study in which cortical dysgenesis was detected in post-mortem brains of mentally handicapped, autistic subjects (Bailey et al.,1998).

Abnormally formed nerve tracts, abnormally migrating 5-HT and catecholaminergic neurons in the hindbrain were also observed to be induced by prenatal VPA exposure, but only in animals exposed to VPA on GD11 exposure. This finding indicates that a critical window must exist for VPA-induced developmental abnormalities in the hindbrain which takes place around the time of neural tube closure. Interestingly, as abnormal tracts running through the pontine tegmentum were reported in
the Bailey et al. (1998) study, this VPA-induced rat model of autism reproduces, at least in part, the pathological findings reported in idiopathic autism.

The present results demonstrate that VPA exposure on GD 9 induced cortical dysgenesis while VPA exposure on GD 11 induced both cortical dysgenesis and abnormal hindbrain development. These findings reveal that the extent of VPA-induced abnormalities varies depending on the timing of exposure to this compound. Further studies on developmental outcomes as a function of the timing of VPA exposure may provide details about why autistic disorders are characterized in terms of a range of indicators rather than a single symptom.

Acknowledgements
This research was supported by a grant for Long-range Research Initiative from the Japan Chemical Industry Association.

References

Arndt, TL, Stodgell, CJ, Rodier, PM. 2005. The teratology of autism. Int J Dev Neurosci 23: 189-199.

Bandim, JM, Ventura, LO, Miller, MT, et al. 2003. Autism and Mobius sequence: an exploratory study of children in northeastern Brazil. Arq Neuropsiquiatr 61: 181-185.

Chess, S. 1971. Autism in children with congenital rubella. J Autism Child Schizophr 1: 33-47.

Ingram, JL, Peckham, SM, Tisdale, B, Rodier, PM. 2000. Prenatal exposure of rats to valproic acid reproduces the cerebellar anomalies associated with autism. Neurotoxicol Teratol 22: 319-324.

Kozma, C. 2001. Valproic acid embryopathy: report of two siblings with further expansion of the phenotypic abnormalities and a review of the literature. Am J Med Genet 98: 168-175.

Moore, SJ, Turnpenny, P, Quinn, A, et al. 2000. A clinical study of 57 children with fetal anticonvulsant syndromes. J Med Genet 37: 489-497.

Nakasato, A, Nakatani, Y, Seki, Y, et al. 2008. Swim stress exaggerates the hyperactive mesocortical dopamine system in a rodent model of autism. Brain Res 1193: 128-135.

Nanson, JL, Hiscock, M. 1990. Attention deficits in children exposed to alcohol prenatally. Alcohol Clin Exp Res 14: 656-661.

Narita, N, Kato, M, Tazoe, M, et al. 2002. Increased monoamine concentration in the brain and blood of fetal thalidomide- and valproic acid-exposed rat: putative animal models for autism. Pediatr Res 52: 576-579.

Ogawa, T, Kuwagata, M, Muneoka, KT, Shioda, S. 2005. Neuropathological examination of fetal rat brain in the 5-bromo-2'-deoxyuridine-induced neurodevelopmental disorder model. Congenit Anom (Kyoto) 45: 14-20.

Rasalam, AD, Hailey, H, Williams, JH, et al. 2005. Characteristics of fetal anticonvulsant syndrome associated autistic disorder. Dev Med Child Neurol 47: 551-555.

Rodier, PM, Ingram, JL, Tisdale, B, Croog, VJ. 1997. Linking etiologies in humans and animal models: studies of autism. Reprod Toxicol 11: 417-422.

Schneider, T, Przewlocki, R. 2005. Behavioral alterations in rats prenatally exposed to valproic acid: animal model of autism. Neuropsychopharmacology 30: 80-89.

Schneider, T, Roman, A, Basta-Kaim, A, et al. 2008. Gender-specific behavioral and immunological alterations in an animal model of autism induced by prenatal exposure to valproic acid. Psychoneuroendocrinology 33: 728-740.

Stanton, ME, Peloso, E, Brown, KL, Rodier, P. 2007. Discrimination learning and reversal of the conditioned eyeblink reflex in a rodent model of autism. Behav Brain Res 176: 133-140.

Stromland, K, Nordin, V, Miller, M, et al. 1994. Autism in thalidomide embryopathy: a population study. Dev Med Child Neurol 36: 351-356.

Tsujino, N, Nakatani, Y, Seki, Y, et al. 2007. Abnormality of circadian rhythm accompanied by an increase in frontal cortex serotonin in animal model of autism. Neurosci Res 57: 289-295.

Sexually dimorphism and social brain circuit: its implication to Autism

Hidenori Yamasue[1,2]*, Nobumasa Kato[2]

[1]Department of Neuropsychiatry, Graduate School of Medicine, University of Tokyo
[2]Department of Psychiatry, Showa University School of Medicine

*To whom correspondence should be addressed at Department of Neuropsychiatry, Graduate School of Medicine, University of Tokyo, 7-3-1 Hongo, Bunkyo-ku, Tokyo 113-8655, Japan.
E-mail: yamasue-tky@umin.ac.jp

Summary. The common features of autism-spectrum disorder (ASD), a highly-heritable pervasive developmental disorder with a significant heterogeneity and multiple-genetic factors, are characterized by severe dysfunction in social reciprocity, abnormalities in social-brain regions, and disproportionately low probability in females. On the other hand, a certain domain of mental function such as emotional memory and social reciprocity shows a significant sex-difference. In addition, recent neuroimaging studies have shown significant sexually-dimorphisms in neuroanatomical correlates of social cognition and behavior. Recently, some sexually-dimorphic factors such as oxytocin have been paid attention because of its possible contribution to mental development especially in social cognitive and behavioral domain. Taken together, it is hypothesized that a sexually-dimorphic factor associating with social function could affect dysfunction in social reciprocity, abnormalities in social-brain regions, and disproportionately low probability in females of ASD. This review article overviewed sexually-dimorphisms in clinical feature of ASD, in normal social cognition, and in social brain function and structure. The association of oxytocin with sexually-dimorphisms, social reciprocity, neural correlates of social congition, and the pathogenesis of ASD were further summarized.

Key Words. Social brain, Sex difference, Neuroimaging, MRI, Autism

1. Sex difference in social cognition

A certain domain of mental function such as social interactive ability and social cognition are sexually-dimorphic in healthy human individuals. In healthy adults, females tend to show strong cooperativeness across nations and cultures (Cloninger et al., 1993; Brandstrom et al., 2001; Farmer et al., 2003), although previous literature showed some inconsistency (Rapoport and Chammah, 1965). Baron-Cohen and his colleagues have revealed sex differences in the several psychometrical measures developed in their research group. Based on the findings, they suggested that the male brain is a defined psychometrically as those individuals in whom systemizing is performed significantly better than empathizing or friendship, and that the female brain is defined as the opposite cognitive profile (Brandstrom et al., 2001; Soderstrom et al., 2002; Baron-Cohen, 2002; Farmer et al., 2003; Baron-Cohen et al., 2003; Baron-Cohen and Wheelwright, 2003; 2004; Lawson et al., 2004; Baron-Cohen et al., 2005).

2. Sex difference in social brain circuit

Regarding neural correlates of social cognition, significant sexually-dimorphisms have also been suggested. Recent functional-imaging studies have reported activations of posterior superior temporal gyrus, posterior inferior frontal gyrus, anterior medial prefrontal cortex, anterior insula, and fusiform gyrus as neural correlates of human social reciprocity and related factors such as empathy, understanding other's emotion, and interpersonal interaction (McCabe et al., 2001; Rilling et al., 2002; Carr et al., 2003; Singer et al., 2004; Decety et al., 2004; Iacoboni et al., 2005). Furthermore, a few studies have suggested sex differences in these activations (Leibenluft et al., 2004; Platek et al., 2005; Azim et al., 2005; Singer et al., 2006). For example, Azim et al. (2005) revealed sex differences in brain activation elicited by humor. While both sexes share the temporal-occipital junction and temporal pole, structures implicated in semantic knowledge and juxtaposition, and the inferior frontal gyrus, likely to be involved in language processing, females activate the left inferior frontal cortex and caudate more than males during comprehension of humor. Platek et al. (2005) also showed sex differences in the neural correlates of perception for child facial resemblance. They showed using functional-Magnetic

Resonance Imaging (f-MRI) that females revealed greater activation in fusiform gyrus to child faces than male when resemblance was not modeled. In contrast, males showed greater cortical activity than females in response to children's faces that resembled themselves. They explained these results with theories of sexual selection. Furthermore, Singer et al. (2006) examined the modulation effect of perceived fairness on brain empathic responses induced by viewing other person's pain measured with f-MRI in males and females separately. Both sexes exhibited empathy-related activation in pain-related brain areas (fronto-insular and anterior cingulate cortices) towards fair person, while these empathy-related responses were significantly reduced in males when observing an unfair person receiving pain. Based on the results, it was suggested that empathic responses are shaped by valuation of other's social behavior, such that they empathize with fair opponents while favouring the physical punishment of unfair opponents.

In addition, sexually-dimorphisms in neuroanatomical substrates of social cognition might be extended at brain structural level. Human altruistic cooperativeness, one of the most important components of our highly organized society is, along with a greatly enlarged brain relative to body size, a spectacular outlier in the animal world. The "social-brain hypothesis" suggests that human brain expansion reflects an increased necessity for information processing to create social reciprocity and cooperation in our complex society. The author's research group reported that the young adult females (n=66) showed greater Cooperativeness as well as larger relative global and regional gray matter volumes than the matched males (n=89), particularly in the social-brain regions including bilateral posterior inferior frontal and left anterior medial prefrontal cortices. Moreover, in females, higher cooperativeness was tightly coupled with the larger relative total gray matter volume and more specifically with the regional gray matter volumes in most of the regions revealing larger in female sex-dimorphism. The global and most of regional correlations between gray matter volumes and Cooperativeness were significantly specific to female (Yamasue et al., 2008). Our results suggest that sexually-dimorphic factors may affect the neurodevelopment of these "social-brain" regions, leading to higher cooperativeness in females.

3. Sexually dimorphism in social brain and autism

Our morphological findings may also have an implication for the pathophysiology of autism-spectrum disorders (ASD); characterized by severe dysfunction in social reciprocity, abnormalities in social-brain, and disproportionately low probability in females (Folstein and Rosen-Sheidley, 2001). Baron-Cohen (2002) proposed the extreme male brain theory of autism that the male brain is a defined psychometrically as those individuals in whom systemizing is performed significantly better than empathizing or friendship, and that the female brain is defined as the opposite cognitive profile (Brandstrom et al., 2001; Soderstrom et al., 2002; Baron-Cohen, 2002; Farmer et al., 2003; Baron-Cohen et al., 2003; Baron-Cohen and Wheelwright, 2003; 2004; Lawson et al., 2004; Baron-Cohen et al., 2005). Using these definitions, autism can be considered as an extreme of the normal male profile. Recently, the hypothesis further suggests that specific aspects of autistic neuroanatomy may also be extremes of typical male neuroanatomy (Baron-Cohen et al., 2005). The our MRI results are consistent with this hypothesis. Previous studies using structural MRI demonstrated smaller anterior cingulate (Haznedar et al., 1997; 2000), superior temporal gyrus, prefrontal cortex (Boddaert et al., 2004; De Fosse et al., 2004; Waiter et al., 2004; McAlonan et al., 2005; Yamasue et al., 2005; Hadjikhani et al., 2006), thalamus (Tsatsanis et al., 2003), posterior inferior frontal gyrus (Hadjikhani et al., 2006) and enlarged amygdala, cerebellum (Howard et al., 2000; Sparks et al., 2002) in subjects with ASD. Our study revealed sex-dimorphism in brain anatomy at a similar location and in the same direction as these previous studies of individuals with autism. Thus, the study may add supportive evidence for Baron-Cohen's extreme male brain theory of autism at the level of brain structure (Yamasue et al., 2008).

4. Sex difference in neural substrates of ASD

Previous studies have repeatedly demonstrated both functional and structural brain abnormalities in individuals with ASD compared with individuals with typical development. Briefly in this section, the previous functional neuroimaging studies, especially indicating abnormalities in so-called social brain regions such as amygdala, fusiform gyrus, medial prefrontal cortices, superior temporal sulcus, and posterior inferior frontal cortices, were overviewed below.

Several previous studies have reported neural substrates of face and gaze processing deficits in individuals with ASD (Schultz et al., 2000; Hubl et al., 2003; Pierce et al., 2001; 2004; 2008; Pelphrey et al., 2005; Dalton et al., 2005; 2007), although the potential confounds have recently been pointed out (Klin 2008). Schultz et al. (2000) reported that the subjects with ASD showed less activation in the fusiform gyrus and greater activation in the right inferior temporal gyrus during face descrimination, the same activation pattern as the controls during object discrimination. Several studies also showed that subjects with ASD fail to activate fusiform face area during a face perception task (Hubl et al., 2003; Pierce et al., 2001). Pierce et al. (2004; 2008) further examined the effect of facial familiarity on the activation of fusiform face area in individuals with ASD. They showed that viewing familiar face such as their mother's face elicited a significant activation in fusiform face area of children with ASD (Pierce et al., 2008) as well as adults with ASD (Pierce et al., 2004). Dalton et al. (2005; 2007) examined the effect of gaze fixation on the aberrant activation in fusiform face area of individuals with ASD or in unaffected siblings of subjects with ASD. Activation in fusiform face area was strongly and positively correlated with the time spent fixating the eyes in the autistic group, suggesting that diminished gaze fixation may account for the fusiform face area hypoactivation to faces previously reported in subjects with ASD (Dalton et al., 2005). Furthermore, the unaffected siblings of subjects with ASD showed the similar pattern to subjects with ASD (Dalton et al., 2007).

Previous studies have suggested that medial prefrontal cortices and cingulate cortices seem to be implicated in the mentalizing and theory of mind, understanding other's intention and emotion (reviewed in Amodio and Frith, 2007). Several studies have reported the contribution of these cortices to the deficits in these interactive processes with others in subjects with ASD (Castelli et al., 2002; Wang et al., 2007). For example, a recent study revealed that subjects with high-functioning ASD showed lesser activation in cingulate cortices during interactive trust-game playing with a human partner than controls (Chiu et al., 2008). The diminished cingulate activation was associated with clinically assessed symptom severity.

Among the temporal cortices engaging in processing multimodal perception such as auditory and visual information, previous studies have suggested superior temporal sulcus processed social perception with other persons such as human voice (e.g. Belin et al., 2000; Grandjean et al., 2005) and biological motion (e.g. Bonda et al., 1996; Grossman et al., 2000; Vaina et al., 2001; Grossman et al., 2002; Pelphrey et al., 2003; Thompson et al., 2005). Individuals with ASD showed dysfunctions in this brain region. Castelli et al. (2002) reported that the healthy adults showed increased activation in a previously reported mentalizing network (medial prefrontal cortex, temporal poles, and superior temporal sulcus ar the temporoparietal junction) during viewing animations of triangles that elicited mentalizing in compared with randomly moving shapes. During the same f-MRI task, the adults with ASD showed less activation than the normal groups in all these regions. Gervais et al. (2004) revealed that subjects with ASD failed to activate superior temporal sulcus voice selective regions in response to vocal sounds, whereas they showed a normal activation pattern in response to nonvocal sounds. It was suggested that abnormal cortical processing of socially relevant auditory information in subjects with ASD. Pelphrey et al. (2005) demonstrated a difference in the response of superior temporal sulcus underlying eye gaze processing in subjects with ASD suggesting that lack of modulation of this brain region by gaze sifts that convey different intentions contributes to the eye gaze processing deficits associated with ASD.

Since superior temporal sulcus, inferior parietal and inferior frontal cortices are implicated in mirroring other's action, these brain regions have recently been thought to be human mirror neuron system (reviewed in Iacoboni and Dapretto, 2006). Several studies have focused on the mirror neuron system as the neural substrates of deficits in social reciprocity of subjects with ASD (Williams et al., 2006; Dapretto et al., 2006). For example, Dapretto et al. (2006) showed that children with autism showed lesser than normal activity in the inferior frontal gyrus (pars opercularis) while imitating and observing emotional expressions. Since the lesser inferior frontal activation was inversely related to symptom severity in the social behavioral domain, it was suggested that a dysfunctional 'mirror neuron system' may underlie the social deficits observed in ASD. Dapretto and colleagues have further examined children with ASD using the f-MRI task to reveal neural correlates of irony comprehension. They showed aberrant activation in inferior frontal gyrus (Wang et al., 2006). Furthermore, a reduced activity in the medial prefrontal cortex and right superior temporal gyrus was observed in children with ASD relative to typical development children during the comprehension of irony. Importantly, a significant group x condition interaction in the medial prefrontal cortex showed that activity was modulated by explicit instructions to attend to facial expression and tone of voice only in the subjects with ASD. Finally, medial prefrontal cortex activity was inversely related to symptom severity in children with ASD such that children with greater social impairment showed less activity in this region (Wang et al., 2007).

5. Conclusion

The currently ongoing evidences overviewed above have revealed that sexually-dimorphic factors implicate in the functional and structural relevance of social brain circuit and in the pathophysiology of ASD. Future study which links the sexually-dimorphic factors with behavioral, brain functional, structural and genetic background of social cognition is expected to uncover the pathophysiology of ASD.

References

Amodio DM, Frith CD (2006) Meeting of minds: the medial frontal cortex and social cognition. Nat Rev Neurosci 7:268-277.

Azim E, Mobbs D, Jo B, Menon V, Reiss AL (2005) Sex differences in brain activation elicited by humor. Proc Natl Acad Sci USA 102:16496-16501.

Baron-Cohen S, Knickmeyer RC, Belmonte MK (2005) Sex differences in the brain: Implications for explaining autism. Science 310:819-823.

Baron-Cohen S, Richler J, Bisarya D, Gurunathan N, Wheelwright S (2003) The systemizing quotient: an investigation of adults with Asperger syndrome or high-functioning autism, and normal sex differences. Philos Trans R Soc Lond B Biol Sci 358:361-374.

Baron-Cohen S, Wheelwright S (2003) The Friendship Questionnaire: an investigation of adults with Asperger syndrome or high-functioning autism, and normal sex differences. J Autism Dev Disord 33:509-517.

Baron-Cohen S, Wheelwright S (2004) The empathy quotient: an investigation of adults with Asperger syndrome or high functioning autism, and normal sex differences. J Autism Dev Disord 34:163-175.

Baron-Cohen S (2002) The extreme male brain theory of autism. Trends Cogn Sci 6:248-254.

Baron-Cohen, S., Richler, J., Bisarya, D., Gurunathan, N., Wheelwright, S (2003) The systemizing quotient: an investigation of adults with Asperger syndrome or high-functioning autism, and normal sex differences. Philos Trans R Soc Lond B Biol Sci 358, 361-374.

Belin P, Zatorre RJ, Lafaille P, Ahad P, Pike B (2000) Voice-selective areas in human auditory cortex. Nature 403:309-312.

Boddaert N, Chabane N, Gervais H, Good CD, Bourgeois M, Plumet MH, Barthelemy C, Mouren MC, Artiges E, Samson Y, Brunelle F, Frackowiak RS, Zilbovicius M (2004) Superior temporal sulcus anatomical abnormalities in childhood autism: a voxel-based morphometry MRI study. Neuroimage 23:364-369.

Bonda E, Petrides M, Ostry D, Evans A (1996) Specific involvement of human parietal systems and the amygdala in the perception of biological motion. J Neurosci 16:3737-3744.

Brandstrom S, Richter J, Przybeck T (2001) Distributions by age and sex of the dimensions of temperament and character inventory in a cross-cultural perspective among Sweden, Germany, and the USA. Psychol Rep 89:747-758.

Carr L, Iacoboni M, Dubeau MC, Mazziotta JC, Lenzi GL (2003) Neural mechanisms of empathy in humans: a relay from neural systems for imitation to limbic areas. Proc Natl Acad Sci USA 100:5497-5502.

Castelli F, Frith C, Happé F, Frith U (2002) Autism, Asperger syndrome and brain mechanisms for the attribution of mental states to animated shapes. Brain 125:1839-1849.

Chiu PH, Kayali MA, Kishida KT, Tomlin D, Klinger LG, Klinger MR, Montague PR (2008) Self responses along cingulate cortex reveal quantitative neural phenotype for high-functioning autism. Neuron 57:463-473.

Cloninger CR, Svrakic DM, Przybeck TR (1993) A psychobiological model of temperament and character. Arch Gen Psychiatry 50:975-990.

Dalton KM, Nacewicz BM, Alexander AL, Davidson RJ (2007) Gaze-fixation, brain activation, and amygdala volume in unaffected siblings of individuals with autism. Biol Psychiatry 61:512-520.

Dalton KM, Nacewicz BM, Johnstone T, Schaefer HS, Gernsbacher MA, Goldsmith HH, Alexander AL, Davidson RJ. (2005) Gaze fixation and the neural circuitry of face processing in autism. Nat Neurosci 8:519-526.

Dapretto M, Davies MS, Pfeifer JH, Scott AA, Sigman M, Bookheimer SY, Iacoboni M (2006) Understanding emotions in others: mirror neuron dysfunction in children with autism spectrum disorders. Nat Neurosci 9:28-30.

De Fosse L, Hodge SM, Makris N, Kennedy DN, Caviness VS Jr, McGrath L, Steele S, Ziegler DA, Herbert MR, Frazier JA, Tager-Flusberg H, Harris GJ (2004) Language-association cortex asymmetry in autism and specific language impairment. Ann Neurol 56:757-766.

Decety J, Jackson PL, Sommerville JA, Chaminade T, Meltzoff AN (2004) The neural bases of cooperation and competition: an fMRI investigation. Neuroimage 23:744-751.

Farmer A, Mahmood A, Redman K, Harris T, Sadler S, McGuffin P (2003) A sib-pair study of the Temperament and Character Inventory scales in major depression. Arch Gen Psychiatry. 60:490-496.

Gervais H, Belin P, Boddaert N, Leboyer M, Coez A, Sfaello I, Barthélémy C, Brunelle F, Samson Y, Zilbovicius M (2004) Abnormal cortical voice processing in autism. Nat Neurosci 7:801-802.

Grandjean D, Sander D, Pourtois G, Schwartz S, Seghier ML, Scherer KR, Vuilleumier P (2005) The voices of wrath: brain responses to angry prosody in meaningless speech. Nat Neurosci 8:145-146.

Grossman E, Donnelly M, Price R, Pickens D, Morgan V, Neighbor G, Blake R (2000) Brain areas involved in perception of biological motion. J Cogn Neurosci 12:711-720.

Grossman ED, Blake R (2002) Brain Areas Active during Visual Perception of Biological Motion. Neuron 35:1167-1175.

Hadjikhani N, Joseph RM, Snyder J, Tager-Flusberg H (2006) Anatomical Differences in the Mirror Neuron System and Social Cognition Network in Autism. Cereb Cortex 16:1276-1282.

Hadjikhani N, Joseph RM, Snyder J, Tager-Flusberg H (2007) Abnormal activation of the social brain during face perception in autism. Hum Brain Mapp 28:441-449.

Haznedar MM, Buchsbaum MS, Metzger M, Solimando A, Spiegel-Cohen J, Hollander E (1997) Anterior cingulate gyrus volume and glucose metabolism in autistic disorder. Am J Psychiatry 154:1047-1050.

Haznedar MM, Buchsbaum MS, Wei TC, Hof PR, Cartwright C, Bienstock CA, Hollander E (2000) Limbic circuitry in patients with autism spectrum disorders studied with positron emission tomography and magnetic resonance imaging. Am J Psychiatry 157:1994-2001.

Hojat M, Gonnella JS, Nasca TJ, Mangione S, Vergare M, Magee M (2002) Physician empathy: definition, components, measurement, and relationship to gender and specialty. Am J Psychiatry 159:1563-1569.

Howard MA, Cowell PE, Boucher J, Broks P, Mayes A, Farrant A, Roberts N (2000) Convergent neuroanatomical and behavioural evidence of an amygdala hypothesis of autism. Neuroreport 11:2931-2935.

Hubl D, Bölte S, Feineis-Matthews S, Lanfermann H, Federspiel A, Strik W, Poustka F, Dierks T (2003) Functional imbalance of visual pathways indicates alternative face processing strategies in autism. Neurology 61:1232-1237.

Iacoboni M, Dapretto M (2006) The mirror neuron system and the consequences of its dysfunction. Nat Rev Neurosci 7:942-951.

Iacoboni M, Molnar-Szakacs I, Gallese V, Buccino G, Mazziotta JC, Rizzolatti G (2005) Grasping the intentions of others with one's own mirror neuron system. PLoS Biol 3:e79.

Kleinhans NM, Richards T, Sterling L, Stegbauer KC, Mahurin R, Johnson LC, Greenson J, Dawson G, Aylward E (2008) Abnormal functional connectivity in autism spectrum disorders during face processing. Brain 131(Pt 4):1000-1012.

Klin A. (2008) Three things to remember if you are a functional magnetic resonance imaging researcher of face processing in autism spectrum disorders. Biol Psychiatry 64:549-551.

Lawson J, Baron-Cohen S, Wheelwright S (2004) Empathising and systemising in adults with and without Asperger Syndrome. J Autism Dev Disord 34:301-310.

Leibenluft E, Gobbini MI, Harrison T, Haxby JV (2004) Mothers' neural activation in response to pictures of their children and other children. Biol Psychiatry 56:225-232.

McAlonan GM, Cheung V, Cheung C, Suckling J, Lam GY, Tai KS, Yip L, Murphy DG, Chua SE (2005) Mapping the brain in autism. A voxel-based MRI study of volumetric differences and intercorrelations in autism. Brain 128:268-276.

McCabe K, Houser D, Ryan L, Smith V, Trouard T (2001) A functional imaging study of cooperation in two-person reciprocal exchange. Proc Natl Acad Sci USA 98:11832-11835.

Pelphrey KA, Mitchell TV, McKeown MJ, Goldstein J, Allison T, McCarthy G (2003) Brain activity evoked by the perception of human walking: controlling for meaningful coherent motion. J Neurosci 23:6819-6825.

Pelphrey KA, Morris JP, McCarthy G (2005) Neural basis of eye gaze processing deficits in autism. Brain 128(Pt 5):1038-1048.

Pierce K, Haist F, Sedaghat F, Courchesne E (2004) The brain response to personally familiar faces in autism: findings of fusiform activity and beyond. Brain 127:2703-2716.

Pierce K, Müller RA, Ambrose J, Allen G, Courchesne E (2001) Face processing occurs outside the fusiform 'face area' in autism: evidence from functional MRI. Brain 124(Pt 10):2059-2073.

Pierce K, Redcay E (2008) Fusiform function in children with an autism spectrum disorder is a matter of "who". Biol Psychiatry 64:552-560.

Platek SM, Keenan JP, Mohamed FB (2005) Sex differences in the neural correlates of child facial resemblance: an event-related fMRI study. Neuroimage 25:1336-1344.

Rapoport A, Chammah AM (1965) Sex differences in factors contributing to the level of cooperation in the prisoner's dilemma game. J Pers Soc Psychol 2:831-838.

Rilling J, Gutman D, Zeh T, Pagnoni G, Berns G, Kilts C (2002) A neural basis for social cooperation. Neuron 35:395-405.

Schultz RT, Gauthier I, Klin A, Fulbright RK, Anderson AW, Volkmar F, Skudlarski P, Lacadie C, Cohen DJ, Gore JC (2000) Abnormal ventral temporal cortical activity during face discrimination among individuals with autism and Asperger syndrome. Arch Gen Psychiatry 57:331-340.

Singer T, Kiebel SJ, Winston JS, Dolan RJ, Frith CD (2004) Brain responses to the acquired moral status of faces. Neuron 41:653-662.

Singer T, Seymour B, O'Doherty JP, Stephan KE, Dolan RJ, Frith CD (2006) Empathic neural responses are modulated by the perceived fairness of others. Nature 439:466-469.

Soderstrom H, Rastam M, Gillberg C (2002) Temperament and character in adults with Asperger syndrome. Autism 6:287-297.

Sparks BF, Friedman SD, Shaw DW, Aylward EH, Echelard D, Artru AA, Maravilla KR, Giedd JN, Munson J, Dawson G, Dager SR (2002) Brain structural abnormalities in young children with autism spectrum disorder. Neurology 59:184-192.

Thompson JC, Clarke M, Stewart T, Puce A (2005) Configural processing of biological motion in human superior temporal sulcus. J Neurosci 25:9059-9066.

Tsatsanis KD, Rourke BP, Klin A, Volkmar FR, Cicchetti D, Schultz RT (2003) Reduced thalamic volume in high-functioning individuals with autism. Biol Psychiatry 53:121-129.

Vaina LM, Solomon J, Chowdhury S, Sinha P, Belliveau JW (2001) Functional neuroanatomy of biological motion perception in humans. Proc Natl Acad Sci USA 98:11656-11661.

Volkmar FR, Szatmari P, Sparrow SS (1993) Sex differences in pervasive developmental disorders. J Autism Dev Disord 23:579-591.

Waiter GD, Williams JH, Murray AD, Gilchrist A, Perrett DI, Whiten A (2004) A voxel-based investigation of brain structure in male adolescents with autistic spectrum disorder. Neuroimage 22:619-625.

Wang AT, Lee SS, Sigman M, Dapretto M (2006) Neural basis of irony comprehension in children with autism: the role of prosody and context. Brain 129:932-943.

Wang AT, Lee SS, Sigman M, Dapretto M (2007) Reading affect in the face and voice: neural correlates of interpreting communicative intent in children and adolescents with autism spectrum disorders. Arch Gen Psychiatry 64:698-708.

Wheelwright S, Baron-Cohen S, Goldenfeld N, Delaney J, Fine D, Smith R, Weil L, Wakabayashi A (2006) Predicting Autism Spectrum Quotient (AQ) from the Systemizing Quotient-Revised (SQ-R) and Empathy Quotient (EQ). Brain Res 1079:47-56.

Williams JH, Waiter GD, Gilchrist A, Perrett DI, Murray AD, Whiten A (2006) Neural mechanisms of imitation and 'mirror neuron' functioning in autistic spectrum disorder. Neuropsychologia 44:610-621.

Yamasue H, Abe O, Suga M, Yamada H, Rogers MA, Aoki S, Kato N, Kasai K (2008) Sex-linked neuroanatomical basis of human altruistic cooperativeness. Cereb Cortex 18:2331-2340.

Yamasue H, Ishijima M, Abe O, Sasaki T, Yamada H, Suga M, Rogers M, Minowa I, Someya R, Kurita H, Aoki S, Kato N, Kasai K (2005) Neuroanatomy in monozygotic twins with Asperger disorder discordant for comorbid depression. Neurology 65:491-492.

Functional Mapping of Sensory and Motor Brain Activity

Stimulating Music: Combining Melodic Intonation Therapy with Transcranial DC Stimulation to Facilitate Speech Recovery after Stroke

Bradley W. Vines[1,2], Andrea C. Norton[1], and Gottfried Schlaug[1]

[1]Department of Neurology, Beth Israel Deaconess Medical Center and Harvard Medical School, 330 Brookline Avenue, Boston, MA, 02215, USA
gschlaug@bidmc.harvard.edu

[2]Current affiliation: Institute of Mental Health, Department of Psychiatry, The University of British Columbia, 430-5950 University Boulevard, Vancouver, BC, V6T 1Z3, Canada
bradley.vines@ubc.ca

Summary. It may be strange to think that singing could help a stroke victim speak again, but this is the goal of Melodic Intonation Therapy (MIT), a speech therapy that emphasizes musical aspects of language. The positive effects of MIT on speech recovery may be mediated by a fronto-temporal brain network in the right hemisphere. We investigated the potential for a non-invasive brain stimulation technique, Transcranial Direct Current Stimulation (tDCS), to augment the benefits of MIT for patients with severe non-fluent aphasias. The tDCS was applied to the posterior inferior frontal gyrus (IFG) of the right hemisphere, under the assumption that the posterior IFG is a key region in the process of recovering from aphasia. The stimulation coincided with an MIT session, conducted by a trained therapist. Participants' language fluency improved significantly more with real tDCS + MIT, compared to sham tDCS + MIT. These results provide evidence that combining tDCS with MIT may enhance activity in a sensorimotor network for articulation in the right hemisphere, to compensate for damaged left-hemisphere language centers.

Key words. Melodic Intonation Therapy, Transcranial Direct Current Stimulation, tDCS, Stroke, Recovery, Neurorehabilitation, Singing, Music Therapy

1 Introduction

Approximately 20% of stroke victims suffer from aphasia, which is a loss of speech and language ability (Schlaug et al., 2008a). Though behavioral therapies for recovery from stroke can have a beneficial effect (Robey, 1994; Holland et al., 1996), recovery is most often incomplete, particularly for patients with large left-hemisphere strokes. Relatively few speech therapy techniques are available to help these patients. An intonation-based speech therapy, Melodic Intonation Therapy, may be particularly suited for patients who suffer from severe non-fluent aphasia (Schlaug et al., 2008a,b). Another line of research has recently emerged which shows that combining behavioral therapies with non-invasive brain-stimulation might enhance the potential for recovery (Schlaug, Renga, Nair, 2008). Indeed, the future of stroke-recovery therapy may lie in *combining* behavioral therapy with complimentary non-invasive brain stimulation to maximally engage brain areas that are important for recovery. We explored this promising frontier of rehabilitation by investigating the effects of combining non-invasive brain stimulation with a behavioral intonation-based speech therapy.

1.1 Aphasia and Music in the Brain

Because some language processes are largely lateralized to the left hemisphere, left-hemisphere damage can lead to devastating forms of aphasia. A stroke affecting the left frontal lobe can cause a non-fluent aphasia with relatively unimpaired comprehension – Broca's aphasia (Luria, 1970). Broca's aphasia hinders the ability to organize elements of speech (e.g., phonemes) into meaningful utterances. Previous research suggests that there are two neural pathways to recovery from Broca's aphasia. One pathway involves the re-activation of peri-lesional cortex in the left hemisphere; generally, this is only possible for patients who have smaller lesions that do not completely destroy Broca's area. The second pathway utilizes the right hemisphere, and may be the only option for patients with large left-hemisphere lesions (Blasi et al., 2002; Mimura et al., 1998; Pizzamiglio et al., 2001; Schlaug et al., 2008b; Thiel et al., 2001; Winhuisen et al., 2005). These studies provide evidence that language-capable centers in the right-hemisphere may compensate for damaged left-hemisphere "eloquent" areas to help patients recover language skill, particularly when damage to the left hemisphere is extensive.

An increasing number of studies point to common neural substrates for language and music (Maess et al., 2001; Koelsch et al., 2002; Patel et al.,

1998, 2003). For example, neuroimaging techniques have revealed both overlapping as well as unique brain networks for speaking and singing (Ozdemir et al., 2006; Brown et al., 2004); though speaking tends to be lateralized to the left hemisphere and singing to the right (Jeffries et al., 2003; Riecker et al., 2000; Sparing et al., 2007), these two behaviors involve some of the same brain areas. In their fMRI study, Ozdemir and colleagues (2006) found that adding speech to melody engaged the right IFG. Singing, or intoned speaking, therefore, may provide a useful means for accessing language-capable brain areas in the right hemisphere for the purpose of facilitating language recovery (Racette et al., 2006).

1.2 Melodic Intonation Therapy

Melodic Intonation Therapy (MIT) is a specialized speech therapy that emphasizes the melodic and rhythmic elements of speech. The technique was inspired by the common clinical observation that severely aphasic patients can sing the lyrics of a song better than they can speak them (Goldstein, 1942; Gerstman, 1964; Geschwind, 1971; Keith & Aronson, 1975; Kinsella et al., 1988; Hebert et al., 2003). MIT uses a simplified and exaggerated prosody in which high probability words and phrases are intoned and tapped out syllable by syllable, with gradually increasing complexity as the patient progresses through levels of difficulty. Research has found MIT to be effective in facilitating significant improvements in language production (Albert et al., 1973; Bonakdarpour et al., 2000; Laughlin et al., 1979; Schlaug et al., 2008a; Sparks et al., 1974; Wilson et al., 2006). MIT's efficacy may be due to its unique potential to engage language-competent brain regions in both hemispheres, and in the right hemisphere in particular (Albert et al., 1973; Schlaug et al., 2008a; Sparks et al., 1974). It is still unknown which brain regions could potentially drive the therapeutic effect of MIT. However, the posterior IFG very likely plays a critical role in the network underlying recovery. It is possible to test the unique contributions of different brain regions by either temporarily blocking them or by enhancing their activity using non-invasive brain-stimulation.

1.3 Transcranial Direct Current Stimulation

Transcranial Direct Current Stimulation (tDCS) is a non-invasive brain stimulation technique that has been shown to influence excitability in a targeted brain region by modulating the spontaneous firing rate of neurons (Priori et al., 1998; Nitsche and Paulus, 2000). Research suggests that the polarity of the current determines the effects of tDCS – anodal tDCS increases cortical excitability and cathodal tDCS decreases excitability. TDCS effects may be mediated by activity in sodium and calcium ion channels as well as by the efficacy of NMDA receptors (Liebetanz et al., 2002; Nitsche et al., 2003a). Anodal tDCS can improve cognitive and behavioral performance on tasks involving the stimulated brain area (Antal et al., 2004; Fregni et al., 2005; Boggio et al., 2006; Kincses et al., 2004; Nitsche et al., 2003b; Vines et al., 2006a). For example, Iyer and colleagues (2005) found that applying anodal tDCS to the left prefrontal cortex significantly improved verbal fluency in healthy participants. Is it possible that tDCS could be used to improve verbal fluency for stroke patients as well?

Transcranial direct current stimulation is an ideal non-invasive brain stimulation technique for use in treatment therapies because it is portable, relatively inexpensive, and safe. Though tDCS does not have the temporal or spatial acuity of Transcranial Magnetic Stimulation (TMS), it is possible to stimulate a larger area of cortex using the technique, and to easily combine tDCS with simultaneous behavioral therapy; this is ideal for modulating cortical activity in a network of related brain areas that is relevant to stroke recovery. The results of studies investigating whether tDCS can be used to improve stroke victims' motor skill have been encouraging (Hesse et al., 2007; Hummel et al., 2005; Hummel et al., 2006; Hummel & Cohen, 2005; Nair et al., 2008; Schlaug et al., 2008c,d). At least one study has investigated the potential for tDCS to facilitate recovery from non-fluent aphasia, with promising results (Monti et al., 2008).

The present study compared the effects of two tDCS conditions (anodal and sham) when applied over right IFG during MIT sessions. We hypothesized that, compared to sham, applying anodal tDCS in coordination with MIT would significantly augment the positive effects of therapy on language production by recruiting music processing in the brain to facilitate speech recovery.

2. Materials and Methods

2.1. Participants

Six adult non-fluent stroke patients participated in the study after giving their informed, written consent following protocol approved by the Beth Israel Deaconess Medical Center IRB. For all participants, at least one year had elapsed since their first ischemic stroke. The participants suffered from

Broca's aphasia due to a stroke affecting the left frontal lobe including the inferior frontal gyrus, with relatively unimpaired comprehension. Prior to this study, they each underwent 75 sessions of Melodic Intonation Therapy as part of a different experimental protocol in the laboratory. The ages of the patient participants ranged between 30 and 81 years. All participants were right handed, except for one who was mixed-handed with a dominant left hand. One of the six participants was bi-lingual - a native Russian speaker with some knowledge of English; the other participants were native English speaking.

2.2. Procedure

Participants underwent two series of three therapy sessions – one session per day - in which tDCS was applied to the right-posterior IFG with an angle towards the temporal lobe during twenty-minutes of MIT administered by a trained therapist. The therapist tailored each MIT session to the level of skill of the participant. For one three-day therapy series, anodal tDCS was applied, and for the other, sham tDCS. The ordering of the two stimulation conditions was counterbalanced across participants such that half of them received the sham tDCS series first. The tDCS was applied for 20-minutes, with the active electrode positioned over participants' right IFG, centered approximately 2.5 centimeters posterior to F8 of the 10-20 International EEG system. The correspondence between F8 and the right IFG has been confirmed by neuroimaging studies (Homan et al., 1987; Okamoto et al., 2004), including our own pilot study using high resolution structural MRI (N=5). We chose to position the active electrode slightly posterior to F8 based upon our pilot study investigating the location of the analogue to Broca's area in the right hemisphere. A number of TMS and tDCS studies have used the 10-20 EEG system to identify the location of brain structures for stimulation (Fregni et al., 2005; Iyer et al., 2005; Kincses et al., 2003; Rogalewski et al., 2004, Vines et al., 2006a,b, 2008a,b). Due to the size of the active electrode (area = 16.3 cm^2), the stimulation may have extended into anterior temporal cortex and ventral premotor cortex, which make up the network of fronto-temporal regions thought to underlie MIT's therapeutic effect. The reference electrode (area = 30 cm^2) was positioned over the left supraorbital region, contralateral to the targeted hemisphere. This location for the reference electrode was functionally ineffective in the experimental design (Nitsche et al., 2003b).

A battery-driven, constant current stimulator (Phoresor, Iomed Inc., Salt Lake City, UT) delivered 1.2 mA of electrical current to a participant's scalp by means of the saline-dampened electrodes. For anodal stimulation, the tDCS current ramped up over the first few seconds, and then remained on for the remainder of the 20-minute stimulation period. The sham control was identical to the anodal stimulation, except that the experimenter reduced the current to zero after it ramped up for 30 seconds; the current then stayed at zero for the remaining time period. Participants reported a tingly or itchy sensation at the start of the stimulation, which typically faded away after a few seconds. This sensation was present for both real and sham tDCS. Gandiga et al. (2006) found that naive participants were not able to distinguish between real and sham tDCS, as employed in a manner similar to the present study. The application of tDCS began five minutes after the start of MIT, and continued five minutes after the end of the MIT session. During the five-minute break after the end of MIT and before the end of the stimulation, the patients rested before completing the verbal fluency tasks.

2.3. Task

Participants were tested on a combined measure of verbal fluency comparing performance on a test-battery before and after each stimulation session. The tasks included automatic production of verbal sequences (e.g., counting from one to twenty-one, pronouncing the days of the week/months of the year, reciting the United States pledge of allegiance, and describing flash-card scenes), as well as picture naming. The flash-card scenes were taken from drawings published with the MIT intervention (Helm-Estabrooks & Albert, 1991). Pictures were drawn from the Snodgrass inventory and the Boston Diagnostic Aphasia Examination (BDAE 2nd edition; Goodglass & Kaplan, 1983). The automatic response items were conducted in the same order for each testing session. Pictures were shown in a new random order for each testing session. The number of items (automatic production and picture naming) depended upon the ability of the participant, and were chosen such that the testing session did not exceed 30 minutes to avoid excessive fatigue for the patients. Patients were instructed to always try their best during each testing session, both pre- and post-therapy; they were blind as to whether they were receiving sham or anodal stimulation.

2.4. Data Analysis

We calculated the dependent variable as the percentage of change in the sum duration of fluency measures from before the first of three stimulation sessions to after the last of three stimulation sessions. This calculation produced two values for each participant: 1. (post anodal series – pre anodal series)/(pre anodal series), 2. (post sham series – pre sham series)/(pre sham series). To ensure equality for all four time-points of interest (pre-anodal, post-anodal, pre-sham, post-sham), the calculation of the dependent variable only included durations for fluency items, or portions there-of, that were intact at all of these time-points. For example, on the task of counting from 1 to 21, if a participant made it to 21 at all measurement points excepting one for which the participant only made it to 18, the duration for counting from 1 to only 18 was used at all time-points. Similarly, only pictures that a participant was able to name at all four time-points of interest were used. Doing this ensured that the material at each time-point was identical in terms of content, or what was actually uttered. The dependent variable, therefore, was not sensitive to changes in the amount of verbal production, but in the rate of verbal production - how quickly the participant was able to speak. The measure reflects fluency, with regard to ease of speech production. The percentage of change found for anodal and sham combined with MIT was compared using a planned two-tailed paired-samples *t*-test.

3 Results

All six participants completed the experimental procedure. Data for the effects of anodal and sham stimulation, combined with MIT, are shown in Figure 1. The *t*-test comparing the effects of anodal and sham tDCS yielded a significant result ($t(5) = 3.22, p = .02$). This result was not due to a significant difference in the pre-stimulation therapy performance. A paired samples *t*-test comparing the pre-anodal duration to the pre-sham duration for each patient did not support abandoning the null hypothesis that the pre-stimulation values were equal in mean ($t(5) = -.31, p = .77$); there was no difference in the pre-stimulation scores for sham and anodal tDCS. Compared to sham tDCS, applying anodal tDCS to the right IFG during MIT produced a significantly greater improvement in verbal fluency.

4 Discussion

The results of this study provide evidence that applying real tDCS during MIT augments the beneficial effects of MIT. By increasing excitability in the right IFG, the anodal tDCS may have increased plasticity in brain areas that are engaged by MIT. We posit that increasing excitability in the right IFG with tDCS enabled greater recruitment of that area of the brain, to facilitate verbal output and fluency.

Future research will investigate whether the positive effects of tDCS were due to the particular placement of the anodal electrode over the right IFG, or if anodal stimulation over other brain areas, such as the right anterior temporal cortex could also improve the beneficial effects of MIT. Additionally, it remains unknown whether tDCS, as applied in this study, exerts a positive influence on language recovery only in combination with a behavioral speech therapy, or if tDCS can be used on its own to improve verbal fluency for stroke patients. Because neural plasticity that facilitates language recovery after stroke may involve the development of neural connections that are latent in the undamaged brain, it is possible that modulating cortical excitability with non-invasive brain stimulation will have its greatest impact when a behavioral therapy is used to induce neuroplastic changes.

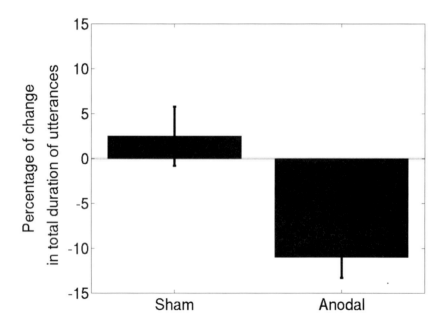

Fig. 1. Data for six Broca's aphasia patient participants. Note that a decrease in the total duration signifies an improvement in verbal fluency. Anodal tDCS led to a significantly greater improvement compared to sham tDCS.

5 Acknowledgments

B.W.V. acknowledges support from the GRAMMY Foundation for this project. This work was also funded by grants from the National Institute of Neurological Disorders and Stroke to B.W.V. (NS053326) and to G.S. (RO1 DC008796). G.S. also acknowledges support from the Mary Crown William Ellis Fund and the Richard Slifka Fund. B.W.V. also acknowledges support from the Michael Smith Foundation for Health Research.

6 References

Albert, M.L., Sparks, R.W., Helm, N.A. (1973). Melodic intonation therapy for aphasia. *Archives of Neurology, 29*,130-131.

Antal, A., Nitsche, M.A., Kruse, W., Kincses, T.Z., Hoffmann, K.-P. et al. (2004). Direct Current Stimulation over V5 Enhances Visuomotor Coordination by Improving Motion Perception in Humans. *Journal of Cognitive Neuroscience, 16* (4), 521–527.

Bangert, M., Peschel, T., Schlaug, G., Rotte, M., Drescher, D. et al. (2006). Shared networks for auditory and motor processing in professional pianists: Evidence from fMRI conjunction. *Neuroimage, 30* (3), 917-926.

Belin, P., Van Eeckhout, P., Zilbovicious, M., Remy, P., Francois, C., et al. (1996). Recovery from non-fluent aphasia after melodic intonation therapy. *Neurology, 47*, 1504–1511.

Blasi, V., Young, A.C., Tansy, A.P., Petersen, S.E., Snyder, A.Z. et al. (2002). Word Retrieval Learning Modulates Right Frontal Cortex in Patients with Left Frontal Damage. *Neuron, 36*, 159–170.

Bonakdarpour, B., Eftekharzadeh, A., Ashayeri, H. (2000). Preliminary report on the effects of melodic intonation therapy in the rehabilitation of Persian aphasic patients. *Iranian Journal of Medical Sciences, 25*, 156-160.

Brown, S., Martinez, M.J., Hodges, D.A., Fox, P.T., Parsons, L.M. (2004). The song system of the human brain. *Cognitive Brain Research, 20* (3), 363-375.

Fregni, F., Boggio, P.S., Nitsche, M., Bermpohl, F., Antal, A. et al. (2005). Anodal transcranial direct current stimulation of prefrontal cortex enhances working memory. *Experimental Brain Research, 166* (1), 23-30.

Gandiga, P.C., Hummel, F.C., Cohen, L.G. (2006). Transcranial DC stimulation (tDCS): A tool for double-blind sham-controlled clinical studies in brain stimulation. *Clinical Neurophysiology, 117* (4), 845-850.

Gerstman, H.L. (1964). A case of aphasia. *Journal of Speech and Hearing Disorders, 29*. 89-91.

Geschwind, N. (1971). Current concepts: aphasia. *New England Journal of Medicine, 284*, 654-656.

Goldstein, K. (1942). *After effects of brain-injuries in war: Their evaluation and treatment.* New York: Grune & Stratton.

Hebert, S., Racette, A., Gagnon, L., Peretz, I. (2003). Revisiting the dissociation between singing and speaking in expressive aphasia. *Brain, 126*, 1-13.

Helm-Estabrooks, N., Albert, M.L. (1991). *Manual of aphasia therapy.* Austin: Pro-Ed.

Hesse, S., Werner, C., Schonhardt, E.M., Bardeleben, A., Jenrich W. et al. (2007). Combined transcranial direct current stimulation and robot-assisted arm training in subacute stroke patients: A pilot study. *Restorative Neurology and Neuroscience, 25* (1), 9-15.

Holland, A.L., Fromm, V., DeRuyter, F., Stein, M. (1996). Treatment efficacy: aphasia. *Journal of Speech and Hearing Research, 39*, S27-S36.

Homan, R.W., Herman, J., Purdy, P. (1987). Cerebral location of international 10-20 system electrode placement. *Electroencephalography and Clinical Neurophysiology, 66*, 376-382.

Hummel, F., Cohen, L.G. (2005). Improvement of motor function with noninvasive cortical stimulation in a patient with chronic stroke. *Neurorehabilitation and Neural Repair, 19* (1), 14-19.

Hummel, F.C., Voller, B., Celnik, P., Floel, A., Giraux, P. et al. (2006). Effects of brain polarization on reaction times and pinch force in chronic stroke. *BMC Neuroscience, 7*: Art. No. 73.

Hummel, F., Celnik, P., Giraux, P., Floel, A., Wu, W.-H., et al. (2005). Effects of non-invasive cortical stimulation on skilled motor function in chronic stroke. *Brain, 128*, 490–499.

Iyer, M.B., Mattu, U., Grafman, J., Lomarev, M., Sato, S. et al. (2005). Safety and cognitive effect of frontal DC brain polarization in healthy individuals. *Neurology 64*, 872–875.

Jeffries, K.J., Fritz, J.B., Braun, A.R. (2003). Words in melody: an H-2 O-15 PET study of brain activation during singing and speaking. *Neuroreport, 14* (5), 749-754.

Keith, R.L., & Aronson, A.E. (1975). Singing as therapy for apraxia of speech and aphasia: report of a case. *Brain and Language, 2*, 483-488.

Kincses, T.Z., Antal, A., Nitsche, M.A., Bartfai, O., Paulus, W. (2004). Facilitation of probabilistic classification learning by transcranial direct current stimulation of the prefrontal cortex in the human. *Neuropsychologia, 42* (1), 113-117.

Kinsella, G., Prior, M.R., Murray, G. (1988). Singing ability after right and left sided brain damage. A research note. *Cortex, 24*, 165-169.

Koelsch, S., Gunter, T.C., von Cramon, D.Y., Zysset, S., Lohmann, G. et al. (2002). Bach speaks: A cortical "language-network" serves the processing of music. *NeuroImage, 17*, 956–966.

Laughlin, S.A., Naeser, M.A. (1979). Effects of three syllable durations using the melodic intonation therapy technique. *Journal of Speech and Hearing Research, 22*, 311-320.

Liebetanz, D., Nitsche, M.A., Tergau, F., Paulus, W. (2002). Pharmacological approach to the mechanisms of transcranial DC-stimulation-induced after-effects of human motor cortex excitability. *Brain, 125*, 2238-2247.

Luria, A.R. (1970). The functional organization of the brain. *Scientific American*, March.
Maess, B., Koelsch, S., Gunter, T.C., Friederici, A.D. (2001). Musical syntax is processed in Broca's area: an MEG study. *Nature Neuroscience, 4* (5), 540-545.
Mimura, M., Kato, M., Sano, Y., Kojima, T., Naeser, M. et al. (1998). Prospective and retrospective studies of recovery in aphasia. Changes in cerebral blood flow and language functions. *Brain, 121,* 2083–94.
Monti, A., Cogiamanian, F., Marceglia, S., Ferrucci, R., Mameli, F. (2008). Improved naming after transcranial direct current stimulation in aphasia. *Journal of Neurology Neurosurgery and Psychiatry, 79* (4), 451-453.
Nair, D.N., Renga, V., Hamelin, S., Pascual-Leone, A., Schlaug, G. (2008). Improving motor function in chronic stroke patients using simultaneous occupational therapy and tDCS. *Stroke, 39* (2), 542.
Nitsche, M.A., Fricke, K., Henschke, U., Schlitterlau, A., Liebetanz, D. et al. (2003a) Pharmacological modulation of cortical excitability shifts induced by transcranial DC stimulation. *Journal of Physiology 553,* 293-301.
Nitsche, M.A., Schauenburg, A., Lang, N., Liebetanz, D., Exner, C. (2003b). Facilitation of implicit motor learning by weak transcranial direct current stimulation of the primary motor cortex in the human. *Journal of Cognitive Neuroscience, 15,* 619-626.
Okamoto, M., Dan, H., Sakamoto, K., Takeo, K., Shimizu, K. et al. (2004). Three-dimensional probabilistic anatomical cranio-cerebral correlation via the international 10–20 system oriented for transcranial functional brain mapping. *Neuroimage, 21,* 99–111.
Ozdemir, E., Norton, A., Schlaug, G. (2006). Shared and distinct neural correlates of singing and speaking. *Neuroimage, 33* (2), 628-635.
Patel A.D. (2003). Language, music, syntax and the brain. *Nature Neuroscience, 6,* 674-681.
Patel, A.D., Gibson, E., Ratner, J., Besson, M., Holcomb, P.J. (1998) Processing syntactic relations in language and music: An event-related potential study. *Journal of Cognitive Neuroscience, 10,* 717-733.
Pizzamiglio, L., Galati, G., Committeri, G.. (2001). The contribution of functional neuroimaging to recovery after brain damage: A review. *Cortex, 37,* 11-31.
Priori, A., Berardelli, A., Rona, S., Accornero, N., Manfredi, M. (1998). Polarization of the human motor cortex through the scalp. *NeuroReport, 9* (10), 2257-2260.
Racette, A., Bard, C., Peretz, I. (2006). Making non-fluent aphasics speak: sing along! *Brain, 129,* 2571-2584.
Riecker, A., Ackermann, H., Wildgruber, D., Dogil, G., Grodd, W. (2000). Opposite hemispheric lateralization effects during speaking and singing at motor cortex, insula and cerebellum. *Neuroreport, 11* (9), 1997-2000.
Robey, R.R. (1994). The efficacy of treatment for aphasic persons: A meta-analysis. *Brain and Language, 47,* 582-608.

Rogalewski, A., Breitenstein, C., Nitsche, M.A., Paulus, W., Knecht, S. (2004). Transcranial direct current stimulation disrupts tactile perception. *European Journal of Neuroscience, 20*, 313-316.

Schlaug, G., Marchina, S., Norton, A. (2008a). From Singing to Speaking: Why singing may lead to recovery of expressive language function in patients with Broca's Aphasia. *Music Perception, 25* (4), 315-323.

Schlaug, G., Norton, A., Marchina, S. (2008b). The role of the right hemisphere in post-stroke language recovery. *Stroke, 39* (2), 542-543.

Schlaug, G., Renga, V., Nair, D. (2008c). Transcranial Direct Current Stimulation in Stroke Recovery. *Archives of Neurology, 65*, 1571-1576.

Schlaug, G., Renga, V. (2008d). Transcranial Direct current stimulation – a non-invasive tool to facilitate stroke recovery. *Expert Review of Medical Devices, 5*, 759-768.

Sparing, R., Meister, I.G., Wienemann, M., Buelte, D., Staedtgen, M. et al. (2007). Task-dependent modulation of functional connectivity between hand motor cortices and neuronal networks underlying language and music: a transcranial magnetic stimulation study in humans. *European Journal of Neuroscience, 25* (1), 319-323.

Sparks, R., Helm, N., Albert, M. (1974). Aphasia rehabilitation resulting from melodic intonation therapy. *Cortex, 10*, 303-316.

Thiel, A., Herholz, K., Koyuncu, A., Ghaemi, M., Kracht, L.W. et al. (2001). Plasticity of Language Networks in Patients with Brain Tumors: A Positron Emission Tomography Activation Study. *Annals of Neurology, 50*, 620–629.

Vines, B.W., Nair, D.G., Schlaug, G. (2006a). Contralateral and ipsilateral motor effects after transcranial direct current stimulation. *Neuroreport, 17* (6), 671-674.

Vines, B.W., Schnider, N., Schlaug, G. (2006b). Testing for causality with tDCS: Pitch memory and the left supramarginal gyrus. *Neuroreport, 17* (10), 1047-1050.

Vines, B.W., Cerruti, C., Schlaug, G. (2008a). Dual-hemisphere tDCS facilitates greater improvements in motor performance compared to uni-hemisphere stimulation. *BMC Neuroscience, 9*, 103.

Vines, B.W., Nair, D.G., Schlaug, G. (2008b). Modulating activity in the motor cortex affects performance for the two hands differently depending upon which hemisphere is stimulated. *European Journal of Neuroscience, 28* (8), 1667-1673.

Wilson, S.J., Parsons, K., Reutens, D.C. (2006). Preserved singing in aphasia: A case study of the efficacy of melodic intonation therapy. *Music Perception, 24* (1), 23-35.

Winhuisen, L., Thiel, A., Schumacher, B., Kessler, J., Rudolf, J. et al. (2005). Role of the Contralateral Inferior Frontal Gyrus in Recovery of Language Function in Post stroke Aphasia: A Combined Repetitive Transcranial Magnetic Stimulation and Positron Emission Tomography Study. *Stroke, 36*, 1759-1763.

Serotonin release acts on 5-HT2 receptors in the dorsomedial medulla oblongata to elicit airway dilation in mice

Mitsuko Kanamaru and Ikuo Homma

Department of Physiology, Showa University School of Medicine, 1-5-8 Hatanodai, Shinagawa-ku, Tokyo 142-8555, Japan
<e-mail> mitsuko@med.showa-u.ac.jp; ihomma@med.showa-u.ac.jp

Summary. Serotonin (5-hydroxytryptamine; 5-HT) excites neurons in the hypoglossal and solitary tract nuclei through 5-hydroxytryptamine 2 (5-HT2) receptors, and contributes to genioglossal muscle activation, hypotension and bradycardia. This study investigated the influence of 5-HT2 receptor-mediated 5-HT action in the hypoglossal and solitary tract nuclei on respiratory variables, particularly airway resistance. Adult male mice were subjected to microdialysis and placed in a double-chamber plethysmograph. 5-HT release and respiratory variables were assessed in response to fluoxetine perfusion or fluoxetine plus LY-53857 coperfusion of the dorsomedial medulla oblongata (DMM), which includes the hypoglossal and solitary tract nuclei. 5-HT release in the DMM was increased but respiratory rate was not affected by fluoxetine perfusion with or without LY-53857. Specific airway resistance was significantly larger with fluoxetine plus LY-53857 coperfusion than at baseline or during perfusion with fluoxetine. Conversely, tidal volume was significantly lower with fluoxetine plus LY-53857-coperfusion than at baseline. These results suggest that 5-HT release in the DMM is regulated by a suppressive effect of local 5-HT transporter activity, which elicits airway dilation and increases tidal volume through local 5-HT2 receptors without affecting respiratory rate.

Key words. Airway resistance, Double-chamber plethysmograph, 5-HT, Hypoglossal nucleus, Microdialysis

1 Introduction

Most patients with obstructive sleep apnea experience upper airway closure in the retropalatal and retroglossal regions. Increased volume of the soft palate, tongue, parapharyngeal fat pads and lateral pharyngeal walls has been demonstrated in these patients (Schwab and Gefter, 2002). During nose breathing, nasal resistance accounts for nearly half of the total airway resistance. During mouth breathing, upper airway resistance (from the mouth, pharynx, glottis, larynx and upper trachea) accounts for a third of the total airway resistance (Ferris et al., 1964). The upper airway is influenced by many dilator muscles (Kubin and Davies, 2002). Further clarifying the control mechanism of airway resistance is important for elucidating the mechanism underlying obstructive sleep apnea.

Several studies have shown the role of serotonin (5-hydroxytryptamine; 5-HT) in the hypoglossal nucleus (nXII) in the activation of the hypoglossal nerve and genioglossal muscle activity, particularly when mediated by 5-HT2 receptors (Kubin et al., 1992; Jelev et al., 2001; Fenik and Veasey, 2003). 5-HT in the nXII modulates genioglossus activity across natural sleep-wake states (Jelev et al., 2001), suggesting that the basal degree of serotonergic activity is important in studying serotonergic physiology.

In the solitary tract nucleus (nTS), 5-HT evokes hypotension and bradycardia (Laguzzi et al., 1984), mediated by 5-HT2 receptors (Merahi et al., 1992). 5-HT2 receptor activity can both excite and inhibit neurons in the nTS (Sévoz-Couche et al., 2000). The nTS is part of the respiratory network, included in the dorsal respiratory group. In mice, afferent convergences in the nTS from pulmonary C-fibers, cardiac receptors, and peripheral chemoreceptors have been shown (Paton, 1998). These findings suggest that 5-HT neurons in the nTS affect respiration.

In the present study, the effects of 5-HT2 receptor activation in the dorsomedial medulla oblongata (DMM), including the nXII and the nTS, on airway resistance and respiratory variables were investigated under local perfusion with fluoxetine, a selective serotonin reuptake inhibitor (SSRI), with or without LY-53857, a 5-HT2 receptor antagonist. 5-HT release was concomitantly measured to confirm 5-HT transporter activity and enhanced-serotonergic transmission in the DMM.

2 Methods

2.1 General

Experiments were performed on 10 male C57BL/6N mice of 10.7 ± 0.8 weeks of age weighing 25.4 ± 0.7 g (mean $\pm$ SEM) (CLEA Japan, Tokyo, Japan). Experiments were approved by the Showa University Animal Experiments Committee. The procedure for surgical implantation of a microdialysis probe in the DMM has been described in detail previously (Kanamaru and Homma, 2007). Briefly, each mouse was anesthetized intraperitoneally with pentobarbital sodium (0.5 mg/0.1 ml saline/10 g body weight). Rectal temperature was kept at 37 °C. The head region was cleaned with an antiseptic, isodine, and locally anesthetized by 2%

xylocaine injection. The medulla oblongata was exposed dorsally. A microdialysis probe (CUP7; membrane length, 1 mm; Carnegie Medicin, Stockholm, Sweden) was ocularly inserted into the medulla oblongata, 0.45 mm lateral, 0.8 mm rostral and 1 mm ventral to the obex. The probe was fixed to the cranial bone with dental cement and the skin incision was closed. Mice were placed in a double-chamber plethysmograph. The microdialysis probe was flushed with artificial cerebrospinal fluid (aCSF; in mM: 121.1 NaCl, 5 KCl, 24 NaHCO$_3$, and 1.5 CaCl$_2$ adjusted to pH 7.4 with 95% O$_2$ and 5% CO$_2$) at 5 µl/min for 40 min and equilibrated at 1.2 µl/min for 80 min. During these periods the mice could recover from the anesthesia and acclimatize to the chamber. Dialysate was collected every 25 min into vials containing 10 µl of 0.02 M acetic acid. Respiratory flow curves for the head and body chambers were plotted with pneumotachographs and pressure transducers (TV-241T and TP-602T, Nihon Kohden) at a 10 kHz sampling rate, and analyzed using PowerLab (ADI Instruments, NSW, Australia). Baseline samples were taken to confirm 5-HT release. After the second baseline sample was taken, the aCSF perfusion was changed to 10^{-5} M fluoxetine (Sigma-Aldrich, St. Louis, MO, USA) or 10^{-5} M fluoxetine plus 10^{-5} M LY-53857 (Sigma-Aldrich).

2.2 5-HT analysis

5-HT concentration was analyzed with an ECD-HPLC (BMA-300; EiCOM, Kyoto Japan) equipped with an EICOMPAK (CA-5ODS 2.1 mm x 150 mm, EiCOM). The mobile phase was sodium phosphate buffer (pH 6.0, 0.1 M) containing 5% methanol, 50 mg/l EDTA·2Na and 100 mg/l sodium pentanesulfonate. The flow rate was 0.23 ml/minute. Column temperature was maintained at 25 °C. 5-HT was oxidized at 400 mV with Ag-AgCl on a graphite electrode. Of each 40-µl sample, 35 µl was injected into the HPLC using an autosampler (NANOSPACE SI-2; Shiseido, Tokyo Japan). Chromatographs were recorded and analyzed with PowerChrom (EPC-300; EiCOM).

2.3 Measurement of specific airway resistance and respiratory variables

Specific airway resistance (sR$_{aw}$) was calculated as: R$_{aw}$ * TGV = tan{2π * (delay time)/(total time)} * (P$_{atm}$-47) * 1.36 * (total time)/2π, where R$_{aw}$ is the airway resistance, TGV is the thoracic gas volume, delay time is the duration between the head and body flows, total time is the duration of one respiratory cycle, and P_{atm} is the ambient pressure (mmHg) (Pennock et al., 1979). Respiratory rate (breaths/min), tidal volume (BTPS; ml/10 g body weight) and minute ventilation (BTPS; ml/10 g body weight) were calculated from the respiratory flow curve for the head chamber calibrated with a 0.5-ml injection of air. The probe sites were verified with 50-μm-thick coronal sections.

2.4 Data analysis

Respiratory variables and sR_{aw} were analyzed for 5 s every 5 min and were averaged for 5 measurements per collection period. 5-HT release and sR_{aw} were expressed as percentages of the mean baseline value. The data were analyzed by one-way repeated-measurement ANOVA, with Greenhouse -Geisser correction (Kanamaru et al., 2001). $P < 0.05$ was considered statistically significant.

3 Results

3.1 5-HT release in the DMM

Baseline 5-HT release in the DMM was the same in both groups (6.76 ± 1.70 fmol/35 μl injection in the fluoxetine group and 5.57 ± 1.49 fmol/35 μl injection in the fluoxetine plus LY-53857 group (n = 5 each)). 5-HT release significantly increased above baseline in both groups (1.9-fold in the fluoxetine group and 2.1-fold in the fluoxetine plus LY-53857 group), but this was not significantly different between the two groups (Fig. 1A).

The microdialysis probe sites were distributed in the DMM, including in the nXII, the nTS, and the dorsal motor nucleus of the vagus, around 7.48 mm posterior to bregma. The locations of probe sites were similar between the fluoxetine and the fluoxetine plus LY-53857 groups (Fig. 1B).

3.2 Specific airway resistance and respiratory variables

sR_{aw} was not significantly affected by fluoxetine, but was significantly increased by 1.9-fold by fluoxetine plus LY-53857 in the fourth collection period. The difference between the two groups was significant (Fig. 2A).

Respiratory rate was not significantly affected by fluoxetine perfusion or fluoxetine plus LY-53857 coperfusion. There was no difference in respiratory rate between the two groups (Fig. 2B).

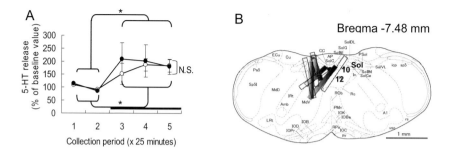

Fig. 1. A: 5-HT release in the DMM in fluoxetine-perfused (open circles, n = 5) and fluoxetine plus LY-53857-coperfused (filled circles, n = 5) groups. Mean ± SEM. The collection period was 25 min.; the drug-perfusion period is indicated by a black bar; *, p < 0.05; N.S., no significance. B: microdialysis probe sites on mouse brain atlas (Franklin and Paxinos, 1997). Open bars, fluoxetine-perfused group; solid bars, fluoxetine plus LY-53857-coperfused group. Sol = solitary tract nucleus; 10 = dorsal motor nucleus of vagus; 12 = hypoglossal nucleus.

Tidal volume was not affected by fluoxetine perfusion into the DMM, but was significantly decreased by fluoxetine plus LY-53857 coperfusion. There was no significant difference between the two groups (Fig. 2 C).

Minute ventilation was obtained by multiplying the respiratory rate with the tidal volume. Minute ventilation tended to decrease during fluoxetine plus LY-53857 coperfusion, but the decrease was not significant. There were no significant differences between the two groups (Fig. 2D).

4 Discussion

In the present study, perfusion of the DMM with fluoxetine, an SSRI, increased local 5-HT release. Perfusion with a 5-HT2 receptor antagonist significantly increased airway resistance and slightly decreased tidal volume without affecting respiratory rhythm. These results suggest that: 1) 5-HT release is regulated by a suppressive effect of local 5-HT transporter activity in the DMM, and 2) the 5-HT release elicits airway dilation and a slight increase in tidal volume by 5-HT2 receptors in the DMM.

5-HT outflow from the hippocampus and frontal cortex of mice is enhanced by systemic administration of fluoxetine, although this is limited by autoreceptors such as 5-HT1A and 5-HT1B (Malagié et al., 2002). There is some evidence that 5-HT transporters are distributed in the nTS, (Huang and Pickel, 2002; Paterson et al., 2004; Nakamoto et al., 2000) and the nXII (Paterson et al., 2004). The present results suggest that the 5-HT dynamics in the DMM are regulated by local 5-HT transporters in mice, i.e. 5-HT transporters take up 5-HT and maintain 5-HT release in the DMM.

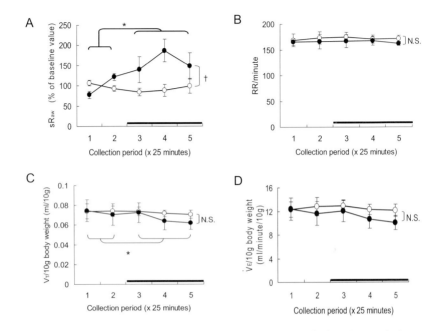

Fig. 2. Respiratory variables obtained for fluoxetine perfusion (open circles, n = 5) and fluoxetine plus LY-53857 coperfusion (filled circles, n = 5) in the DMM. A: specific airway resistance (sR$_{aw}$). B: respiratory rate (RR). C: tidal volume (V$_T$). D: minute ventilation ($\dot{V}_E$). Mean $\pm$ SEM. The drug-perfusion period is indicated by a black bar; *, $p < 0.05$; †, $p < 0.05$; N.S., no significance.

Similar increases in 5-HT release during fluoxetine perfusion and fluoxetine plus LY-53857 coperfusion demonstrate similar degrees of serotonergic stimulation. Therefore, the different responses with and without a 5-HT2 receptor antagonist depend on different activity levels of the 5-HT2 receptors, not the serotonergic neurons.

In this study, a microdialysis probe for the DMM was ocularly inserted to a depth of 1 mm from the dorsal surface of the medulla oblongata at the level of the area postrema. Only a membrane of the probe was inserted into the brain, which minimized brain damage and raised the accuracy of the probe position. However, there was some difficulty in rigid fixation of the probe onto the cranial bones and in free movement of neck. Therefore, acute experiments were performed.

5-HT perfusion of the nXII increases sleeping genioglossal muscle activity to normal waking levels in rats (Jelev et al., 2001). Hypoglossal motoneurons in cats and hypoglossal nerve activity in rats are stimulated by 5-HT2 receptors in the nXII (Kubin et al., 1992; Fenik and Veasey, 2003). Paroxetine, an SSRI, augments genioglossal electromyographic activity in normal humans (Sunderram et al., 2000). Some SSRIs decrease the apnea-hypopnea index during REM sleep in obstructive sleep apnea patients (Hanzel et al., 1991; Kraiczi et al., 1999). In the present study, 5-HT2 receptor-mediated 5-HT activity in the DMM decreased airway resistance, suggesting that 5-HT2 receptor activity in the nXII excites the hypoglossal nerve, contracts the genioglossal muscle, and elicits airway dilation.

During REM sleep, airflow resistance above the larynx is twice as high as during wakefulness in normal humans (Hudgel et al., 1984). In our study, the sR_{aw} with a SSRI and a 5-HT2 receptor antagonist was twice as high as during stimulation by an SSRI alone. This suggests that airway dilation is functionally influenced by 5-HT2 receptor activity in the nXII.

In vagotomized and anesthetized rats, the contribution of serotonergic receptors in the nXII to hypoglossal nerve activity is 35% (Fenik et al., 2005) and to genioglossal muscle activity is 50% (Sood et al., 2005). This was similar to the degree of 5-HT2 receptor contribution to airway resistance in our experiments. The serotonergic drive modulating genioglossal muscle activity, however, was little observed in vagi-intact rats (Sood et al., 2005), which indicates that a minimal endogenous 5-HT drive in the nXII modulates genioglossal muscle activity in rats unless augmented by neural input. Further experiments are needed to clarify the physiological conditions activating serotonergic input to the nXII.

Tidal volume was significantly decreased by fluoxetine plus LY-53857 coperfusion, but the effect was not statistically different from the effect of fluoxetine perfusion alone. Thus manipulation of only 5-HT2 receptors in the DMM has a minor effect on the regulation of tidal volume.

Respiratory rhythm generator is distributed throughout the ventral respiratory group (Ballanyi et al., 1999; Onimaru and Homma, 2003). Stimulation of 5-HT2 receptors in the DMM of resting mice may not affect the respiratory rhythm generators.

The increase in 5-HT release during fluoxetine perfusion did not affect sR_{aw} and tidal volume. Hypoglossal 5-HT decreases glutamate release from the raphe pallidus to the nXII through presynaptic 5-HT1A or 1B receptors (Bouryi and Lewis, 2003). This suggests that spontaneous 5-HT release in the DMM has already elicited airway dilation and increased tidal volume before fluoxetine perfusion; stimulates the inhibitory 5-HT1A and 5-HT1B receptors and excitatory 5-HT2 receptors; or both.

In conclusion, 5-HT release in the DMM is regulated by a suppressive effect of local 5-HT transporters. The 5-HT release in the DMM elicits airway dilation and a slight increase in tidal volume without affecting respiratory rhythm. Those effects are mediated by 5-HT2 receptors. The inactivation of 5-HT2 receptor activity in the DMM doubles the airway resistance. It is useful to measure airway resistance for elucidation of mechanisms underlying upper airway control and obstructive sleep apnea.

References

Ballanyi K, Onimaru H, Homma I (1999) Respiratory network function in the isolated brainstem-spinal cord of newborn rats. Prog Neurobiol 59:583-634

Bouryi VA, Lewis DI (2003) The modulation by 5-HT of glutamatergic inputs from the raphe pallidus to rat hypoglossal motoneurones, in vitro. J Physiol 553:1019-1031

Fenik P, Veasey SC (2003) Pharmacological characterization of serotonergic receptor activity in the hypoglossal nucleus. Am J Respir Crit Care Med 167:563-569

Fenik VB, Davies RO, Kubin L (2005) REM sleep-like atonia of hypoglossal (XII) motoneurons is caused by loss of noradrenergic and serotonergic Inputs. Am J Respir Crit Care Med 172:1322-1330

Ferris BG., Mead J, Opie LH (1964) Partitioning of respiratory flow resistance in man. J Appl Physiol 19:653-658

Franklin KBJ, Paxinos G (1997) The mouse brain in stereotaxic coordinates. Academic Press Inc, California

Hanzel DA, Proia NG, Hudgel DW (1991) Response of obstructive sleep apnea to fluoxetine and protriptyline. Chest 100:416-421

Huang J, Pickel VM (2002) Serotonin transporters (SERTs) within the rat nucleus of the solitary tract: subcellular distribution and relation to 5HT2A receptors. J Neurocytol 31:667-679

Hudgel DW, Martin RJ, Johnson B, Hill P (1984) Mechanics of the respiratory system and breathing pattern during sleep in normal humans. J Appl Physiol 56:133-137

Jelev A, Sood S, Liu H, Nolan P, Horner RL (2001) Microdialysis perfusion of 5-HT into hypoglossal motor nucleus differentially modulates genioglossus activity across natural sleep-wake states in rats. J Physiol 532:467-481

Kanamaru M, Iwase M, Homma I (2001) Neuronal histamine release elicited by hyperthermia mediates tracheal dilation and pressor response. Am J Physiol Regul Integr Comp Physiol 280:R1748-1754

Kanamaru M, Homma I (2007) Compensatory airway dilation and additive ventilatory augmentation mediated by dorsomedial medullary 5-hydroxytryptamine 2 receptor activity and hypercapnia. Am J Physiol Regul Integr Comp Physiol 293:R854-860

Kraiczi H, Hedner J, Dahlöf P, Ejnell H, Carlson J (1999) Effect of serotonin uptake inhibition on breathing during sleep and daytime symptoms in obstructive sleep apnea. Sleep 22:61-67

Kubin L, Tojima H, Davies RO, Pack AI (1992) Serotonergic excitatory drive to hypoglossal motoneurons in the decerebrate cat. Neurosci Lett 139:243-248

Kubin L, Davies RO (2002) Mechanisms of Airway Hypotonia. In: Pack AI (ed) Lung biology in health and disease, Vol 166, Sleep apnea. Marcel Dekker, New York, pp99-154

Laguzzi R, Reis DJ, Talman WT (1984) Modulation of cardiovascular and electrocortical activity through serotonergic mechanisms in the nucleus tractus solitarius of the rat. Brain Res 304:321-328

Malagié I, David DJ, Jolliet P, Hen R, Bourin M, Gardier AM (2002) Improved efficacy of fluoxetine in increasing hippocampal 5-hydroxytryptamine outflow in 5-HT1B receptor knock-out mice. Eur J Pharmacol 443:99-104

Merahi N, Orer HS, Laguzzi R (1992) 5-HT2 receptors in the nucleus tractus solitarius: characterisation and role in cardiovascular regulation in the rat. Brain Res 575:74-78

Nakamoto H, Soeda Y, Takami S, Minami M, Satoh M (2000) Localization of calcitonin receptor mRNA in the mouse brain: coexistence with serotonin transporter mRNA. Mol Brain Res 76:93-102

Onimaru H, Homma I (2003) A novel functional neuron group for respiratory rhythm generation in the ventral medulla. J Neurosci 23:1478-1486

Paterson DS, Belliveau RA, Trachtenberg F, Kinney HC (2004) Differential development of 5-HT receptor and the serotonin transporter binding in the human infant medulla. J Comp Neurol 472:221-231

Paton JF (1998) Pattern of cardiorespiratory afferent convergence to solitary tract neurons driven by pulmonary vagal C-fiber stimulation in the mouse. J Neurophysiol 79:2365-2373

Pennock BE, Cox CP, Rogers RM, Cain WA, Wells JH (1979) A noninvasive technique for measurement of changes in specific airway resistance. J Appl Physiol 46:399-406

Schwab RJ, Gefter WB (2002) Anatomical Factors. Insights from Imaging Studies. In: Pack AI (ed) Lung Biology in Health and Disease, Vol 166, Sleep Apnea. Marcel Dekker, New York, pp1-30

Sévoz-Couche C, Wang Y, Ramage AG, Spyer KM, Jordan D (2000) In vivo modulation of nucleus tractus solitarius (NTS) neurons by activation of 5-hydroxytryptamine 2 receptors in rats. Neuropharmacology 39:2006-2016

Sood S, Morrison JL, Liu H, Horner RL (2005) Role of endogenous serotonin in modulating genioglossus muscle activity in awake and sleeping rats. Am J Respir Crit Care Med 17:1338-1347

Sunderram J, Parisi RA, Strobel RJ (2000) Serotonergic stimulation of the genioglossus and the response to nasal continuous positive airway pressure. Am J Respir Crit Care Med 161:925-929

Breathing is to live, to smell and to feel

Yuri Masaoka, Ikuo Homma

Department of Physiology II, Showa University School of Medicine, 1-5-8 Hatanodai, Shinagawa-ku, Tokyo 142-8555, Japan
<e-mail>faustus@med.showa-u.ac.jp

Summary. Previously we tested simultaneous recordings of electroencephalograms and respiration in normal subjects during threshold and recognition levels of olfaction. The study identified changes of respiratory pattern during odor stimuli and found that inspiratory phase-locked alpha oscillation (I-α) from the averaged potentials were triggered by inspiration onset. We performed dipole analysis of I-α and found the dipoles were located in the olfactory-related areas: the entorhinal cortex, hippocampus, amygdala, and the orbitofrontal cortex. As we often experienced that olfaction is habituated with constant exposure of odor presentation, we compared the respiratory patterns, I-α, and dipole localizations of I-α during recognition of odor with those of adaptation in odor. We found that changes in tidal volume and respiratory rate returned to the normal breathing level during the adaptation period. From averaging EEGs triggered as the inspiration onset, I-α was observed in all electrodes positions during perception of odor; on the other hand, power spectra of frontal areas decreased during the adaptation period. During the adaptation period, dipoles were not estimated in the orbitofrontal cortex, but sustained activations in the entorhinal cortex and hippocampus were observed.

Key words. EEG, dipole tracing method, olfaction, respiration, adaptation, limbic system

1 Introduction

Neuroimaging studies using positron emission tomography (PET) and functional magnetic resonance imaging (fMRI) have revealed olfactory brain regions which relate higher olfactory processing such as discrimination (Rolls et al. 2003), imagination and memory (Levy et al. 1999), and emotion (Royet et al. 2000). These neuroimaging studies have provided information regarding the areas related to olfaction; however, these data lack the assumption that olfaction is largely depended on respiratory activities. Perception and emotion of olfaction are largely dependent on inspiration; we are able to smell through inspiring. Previously we tested simultaneous recordings of electroencephalograms (EEG) and respiration in normal subjects during threshold and recognition levels of olfaction (Masaoka and Homma, 2005). The study identified changes of respiratory pattern during odor stimuli and found that inspiratory phase-locked alpha oscillation (I-α) from the averaged potentials triggered as the inspiration onset. The EEG dipole tracing method (Homma et al, 2001; Okamoto and Homma, 2004) which estimates the active area of the brain, referred to as a dipole location, from the surface potentials. We found that the dipoles were located in the olfactory-related areas: the entorhinal cortex (ENT), hippocampus (HI), amygdala (AMG), and the orbitofrontal cortex (OFC). We suggested that I-α occurred during olfactory stimuli may originate from these olfactory-related areas, and these oscillations were phase-locked to inspiration. These results obtained in the previous study focused on the respiratory pattern, I-α and I-α related olfactory limbic areas without habituation of odors; namely, we paid careful attention to avoid adaptation of odor in all subjects.

We often experience that olfaction is habituated with constant exposure of odor presentation (Ekman et al, 1967). Three factors seem to cause the adaptation in odor. One is the olfactory receptor level (Kurahashi and Menini, 1997), the second is the level of the olfactory bulbs (Shipley and Ennis, 1996), and the last is the primary olfactory cortex the piriform cortex (Pir) (Wilson, 1998).

Previously a fMRI study reported that habituation in olfaction appeared to be caused by not only the olfactory receptor level but also olfactory central structures (Poellinger at al. 2004). In this study, we compared the respiratory patterns, I-α, and dipole localizations of I-α during recognition of odor with those of adaptation in odor. We hypothesized that if odor recognition and odor-induced feeling were involved in the activation of OFG, frontal areas of I-α oscillation might be suppressed and dipoles in the OFC areas would disappear during the adaptation of odor.

2 Method

Five right-handed men (mean age 29.5.6±10.7 years) participated in this study. Subjects with asthma or any allergy were excluded. All subjects completed the the odor detection acuity, and odor recognition acuity were evaluated in all subjects by means of T&T olfactometer (Takasuna Co., LTD, Tokyo, Japan) prior to the experiments. The olfactometer is used with five odors (odor A, β-phenyl ethyl alcohol; odor B, methyl cyclopentenolone; odor C, iso-valeric acid; odor D, γ-undecalactone; odor E, skatole), each at eight different concentrations (-2 to +5). All subjects were normal to detect and recognize the odors. A detailed description about the olfactory test has been reported elsewhere (Masaoka et al. 2005).

2.1 Recordings of the EEG and respiration.

Twenty-one electrodes were attached according to the International 10-20 system, with the reference electrode on the right earlobe. An EEG and electro-oculogram were recorded and stored in a digital EEG analyzer (DAE-2100, Nihon Kohden, Tokyo, Japan). The EEG was sampled at 1000HZ through a 0.016 to 30Hz bandpass filter. Impedances were kept below 10KΩ. The subject put on a facemask with a transducer connected to a respiratory monitor (Aeromoniter AE280, Minato Medical Science, Osaka, Japan) for measurement of respiratory pattern and metabolism. The respiratory monitor calculated breath-by-breath minute ventilation ($\dot{V}_E$), tidal volume (V_T), respiratory frequency (fR), O_2 consumption ($\dot{V}O_2$), end-tidal CO2 (FETCO$_2$). Respiratory flow data obtained with the respiratory monitor were also stored in the EEG analyzer. Since we assume that the perception and sensation of smell are dependent on inspiring, the onset of inspiration was used as a trigger for averaging potentials. All sniffing activities were excluded from the averaging. Eye blinks or artifactual activity exceeding ±50μv were excluded.

2.2 Stimuli presentation

Since all subjects reported that odor D (γ-undecalactone) was the most pleasant in the olfactory test, in this study we used γ-undecalactone of each subject's recognition level for the stimuli. We asked subjects how they feel about the odors by visual analogue scale (VAS) every 15 s (maximum right: smell very strong, maximum left: smell nothing). Adaptation toward odor was defined when the subjects indicated "smell nothing" on the VAS. EEG averages were divided into "odor stimulation", which means subject can recognize or feel the odor, and "adaptation", which indicates subjects feel nothing toward the odor stimuli. Respiratory flow and averaging EEG divided into odor stimulation period and adaptation period are indicated in the Figure 1.

2.3 Data analysis

Respiratory variables

All statistical analyses were performed with a commercially available statistical package (SPSS, Ver. 11.0; SPSS, Tokyo, Japan). Each respiratory variable during the rest, odor stimuli and adaptation were analyzed with one-way repeated measures analysis of variance (ANOVA). Greenhouse-Geisser adjustment of the degrees of freedom was applied to the ANOVA analysis to correct for violation of the assumption of sphericity. Post-hoc tests were performed with Bonferroni tests.

EEG powers of band component

EEG power according to the alpha component of each electrode position was calculated from the inspiratory triggered averaged potential from each subject. Spectral power was analyzed by fast fourier transformation (spectral analysis) using EEG analysis software EEG Focus (Version 2.1.,Nihon Koden). Data indicates mean alpha power from all subjects.

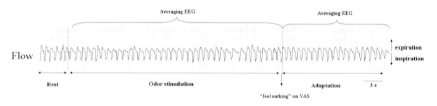

Fig. 1. Respiratory flow during rest, odor stimulation and adaptation. Adaptation toward odor was defined when the subjects indicated "smell nothing" on the VAS. EEG averages were divided into "odor stimulation", which means subject can recognize or feel the odor, and "adaptation", which indicates subjects feel nothing toward the odor stimuli. Respiratory flow and averaging EEG divided into odor stimulation period and adaptation period.

Dipole analysis

Potentials were averaged on the EEG analyzer and the data of averaged potentials transferred to the software of the EEG dipole tracing method of a scalp-skull-brain head model (SSB/DT)(Bs-navi, Brain research and development). Detailed descriptions of the SSB/DT method (Brain Space Navigator, BS-navi, Brain Research and Development, Japan) have been reported elsewhere (Homma et al., 2001; Masaoka et al., 2005; Inoe et al., 2008). SSB/DT calculates the source generators in the brain from the evoked potential by fitting a mathematical model of assumed equivalent dipoles to the data actually recorded from the surface of the scalp. The actual potentials actually recorded from 21 electrodes (Vmeas) are compared with the calculated potential distribution from 2 equivalent current dipoles (Vcal), and the locations of dipoles and vector moments are determined if the square differences between Vmea and Vcal re at a minimum. Root-mean-square (RMS) quality of fit was indicated as dipolarity %. Goodness to fit of more than 98% was considered as significant. Since dipole localization from the grand averaged potential across all subjects with the MNI model showed typical regions for the event because the S/N ratio was increased (Inoue et al., 2008), dipole estimations from the grand averaged potential across all subjects during odor stimuli (not adaptation period) and adaptation were performed.

3 Results

Table 1 shows $\dot{V}_E$, V_T, fR, $ETCO_2$ and $\dot{V}O_2$ during the rest, odor stimulation and adaptation periods. No changes in $\dot{V}O_2$ were observed throughout the experiment (P>0.05). V_T and fR were changed during odor stimulation (P<0.05). Uunchanged $\dot{V}O_2$ means that these respiratory changes were not altered by meeting metabolic requirements (P>0.05). $ETCO_2$ were also unchanged during odor stimulation and adaptation periods (P>0.05).

V_T increased and fR decreased during odor stimulation, but these changes were back to the normal resting level during adaptation. $\dot{V}_E$, were constantly unchanged throughout the recordings (P>0.05).

Figure 2 shows the averaged potentials triggered by the onset of inspiration during odor stimulation (left) and adaptation (right). Each electrode's mean power spectral of alpha bands from all subjects is illustrated as bar graphs.

Table 1. Effect of odor stimulation and odor-induced adaptation on respiratoy parameters.

	Baseline	Odor stimulation	Adaptation
$\dot{V}_E$ (l)	7.5±0.9	7.5±0.2	7.9±0.5
V_T (ml)	563±24	715±112 **	573±25
RR(breath/min)	13.3±1.5	10.7±1.9 *	13.6±0.5
$ETCO_2$ (%)	5.63±0.3	5.75±0.49	5.5±0.2
$\dot{V}O_2$(ml)	228±13	230±10	235±9.8

* $P<0.05$

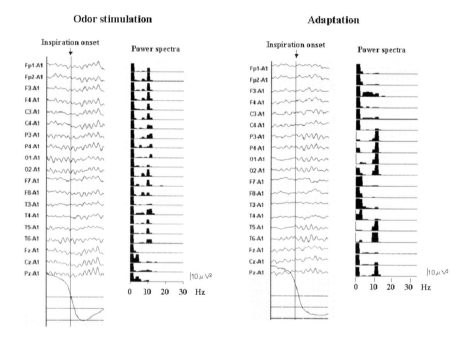

Fig.2 Averaged potentials triggered by the onset of inspiration during odor stimulation (left) and adaptation (right). Each electrode's mean power spectral of alpha bands from all subjects is illustrated as bar graphs.

The alpha rhythm is a waveform with a characteristic 8-12Hz frequency. As observed in Figure 2, the waveforms are categorized as alpha band oscillations, and these waves were synchronized with inspiration for electrode positions during odor stimulation (left). However, during adaptations, I-α were not observed in all electrodes except P3, P4, O1, O2, T5 and T6. Alpha rhythms were often observed on the parietal and occipital areas in the averaged potentials triggered as inspiration onset during the rest (Masaoka and Homma, 2005); however, during the adaptation, temporal areas of T5 and T6 were still locked to inspiration. Results of dipole analysis are shown in Figure 3. During odor stimulation, dipoles were located in the right ENT at 50 ms, in the left OFG at 200 ms. Finally, from 350ms to 400 ms, dipoles were located in the right ENT, AMG, HI and the left OFC. A previous study suggested that odor identification or feeling toward odor could be recognized during 300 ms and 400 ms (Masaoka and Homma, 2005). On the other hand, during the adaptation period, dipoles were found in the left ENT and HI at 120 ms. These areas of dipoles were constantly observed until 400 ms.

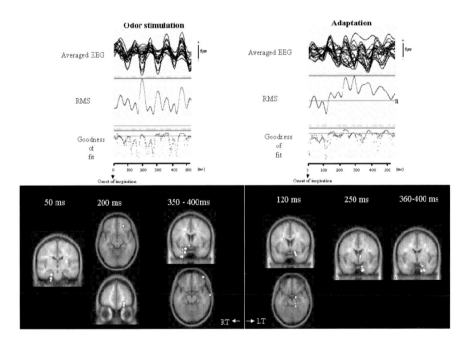

Fig.3 Results of dipole analysis during odor stimulation and adaptation period. Refer to color plates.

4 Discussion

In this study, we investigated the respiratory pattern, I-α and dipole localization of I-α during odor stimulation and an odor-induced adaptation period. We found that changes in V_T, and fR were back to the normal breathing level during the adaptation period. From the observation of averaging EEGs triggered as the inspiration onset, I-α was observed in all electrode positions during perception of odor; on the other hand, power spectra of frontal areas were decreased during the adaptation period. During the adaptation period, dipoles were not estimated in the OFC, but sustained activations in the ENT and HI were observed.

4.1 Olfaction and respiration

Various sensory stimulation such as visual and audition produce emotions. Odors have the strong potential to induce memories and emotions more than other sensory modalities. The process of olfaction is different from the visual, auditory, gestation and somatosensation. Olfactory information progresses directly from the olfactory receptors in the nasal mucosa to the olfactory bulbs and from the olfactory bulbs to the olfactory limbic areas without relaying through the thalamus. Olfaction is the main input for producing cognition and emotions in animals because primates need rapid evaluation of environmental danger, identification of food or recognition of sex differences through the olfactory system, all of which enhance immediate responses toward impending events. Animal studies have characterized the process of odor information. A signal from the olfactory bulbs transmit to the prepiriform and the Pir as a primary olfactory cortex; other targets are the anterior olfactory nucleus, AMG, olfactory tubercle and the ENT. These targeted areas are converged to the OFC which is responsible for a higher order such as olfactory discrimination and feeling. These areas related to olfaction have also been confirmed the neuroimaging studies in humans (Sobel et al., 1998; Royet et al., 2000; Rolls et al., 2001; Masaoka et al., 2005).

It is important to know that perception of odor is dependent on respiratory activities; our sense of smell is enhanced by inspiration. We detected the process of olfaction using the dipole tracing analysis and dipole locations in the ENT (a part of the Pir), HI, AMG and OFG in a millisecond range from the inspiration onset (Masaoka and Homma, 2005). Every inspiration including an odor molecule activates the primary olfactory cortex, and olfactory-related limbic areas, as well as the areas related to the cognition and emotions.

4.2 Respiration, emotion and adaptation in olfaction.

By inspiring, direct stimulation of the olfactory limbic areas unconsciously alters the respiratory pattern. Unpleasant odors increase respiratory rates and induce rapid shallow breathing patterns, and pleasant odors induce deep breathing (Masaoka and Homma, 2005). Not only the olfaction but also respiration is altered by emotions (Boiten et al., 1994). There is direct evidence that stimulation of the AMG, the center of emotion, causes an increase in respiratory rate (Masaoka and Homma, 2004). Respiratory activity is regulated in the brainstem for metabolic purpose; however, stimulation of the higher structure, especially the AMG, has a dominant effect on the respiratory pattern. In this study, we confirmed that V_T increased and fR decreased during the pleasant olfactory stimulus, showing the deep and slow breathing. We found that these respiratory changes were returned to the normal breathing during adaptation.

This indicates that subject felt nothing toward odor; in other words, if we observe the respiratory pattern, we can understand objectively whether the subject is habituated odor or not. From the point of brain activations, Poellinger et al. reported that activities of the Pir and HI were decreased, showing habituation during prolonged olfactory stimulation.

It is interesting that our results show that respiratory changes observed during the perception of odor returned to the normal breathing during adaptation period but the dipole results show the sustained dipoles localized in the ENT and HI. If these areas remained activated, respiration might show the same pattern observed in the perception of odor. We will discuss this theme in later sections.

4.3 OFC and the habituation in olfaction.

The role of the OFC in olfaction has been reported for recognition, identification and emotional feeling. These might be a higher order of olfactory function. Our previous study (Masaoka and Homma, 2005) suggested that activations of the OFC at 300 ms to 400 ms from inspiration onset are for recognition including identification and perception of feeling of odors. Dipoles were not estimated in the OFC in patients with Parkinson's disease (PD) who had impaired recognition of odor (Masaoka et al., 2006). PD patients had impaired odor recognition as well as a low emotional response toward odor. The study concluded that weak activation of OFC in PD patients could be caused by low activations in the ENT, HI and AMG. Pathological changes of these areas might be a factor causing low activation of OFC. Therefore, activation of OFC is need for recognition and emotion through the activation of primary and limbic olfactory structures.

In this study, we found no activations in the OFC during the adaptation period. It is reasonable to say that activations of OFC were observed when the subject recognized the odor and disappeared when subjects were adapted and felt nothing toward the odor. In addition to results of dipole analysis, I-α of frontal areas were decreased during the adaptation period, which means that I-α including the frontal areas might be related to recognition, identification and odor induced-feeling. This result could prove that frontal areas and OFC play a role of recognition and emotional perception for odors.

4.4 Adaptation of pleasant odor and OFC.

We have reported that an unpleasant odor increases respiratory rate with rapid and shallow breathing, and a pleasant odor decreases respiratory rate with slow and deep breathing (Masaokaet al., and Homma, 2005, 2006). Not only the unpleasant olfactory stimuli but also negative emotions such as fear and anxiety cause an increase in respiratory rate. The AMG has a role of emotions, especially fear and anxiety in animal and humans (Davis, 1992). Electrical stimulation on the AMG causes an increase in respiratory rate. These studies proved that the limbic areas including the AMG are important for emotion, especially the negative emotions and physiological responses. It could be assumed that it is hard to identify the areas related to pleasant emotions because pleasant feelings are largely dependent on individuals' memories and experiences. Our previous study concluded that a pleasant feeling toward odor is a higher function compared with negative emotions of odor because pleasant emotions might include a feeling of motivation, intention and attention. This conclusion is drawn from the observation of respiratory pattern and brain activity in our previous two studies (Masaoka and Homma, 2005; Masaoka et al. 2006). Both unpleasant and pleasant odors activate ENT, HI, AMG and OFC in accordance with the inspiration onset. However, activation of the AMG from unpleasant odor stimuli is stronger than that of a pleasant odor. A pleasant odor activates the prefrontal and the premotor areas. These areas of activation might include motivation, intention and attention which are related to the desire and inspire and control of breathing. Another study also suggested that a pleasant sensation caused by odor needs strong activation of the limbic structures; these areas of activation caused by a pleasant odor (including evaluation) have to rely on a higher function such as decision and motivation. Strong activation of the limbic areas might be decreased by adapting process or by inhibitory process of the higher cortical areas. Deep and slow breathing, observed during a pleasant odor, might be the phenomenon showing a higher role of emotional responses and hence that need to control breathing based on the activations of the limbic areas.

Poellinger et al. suggested that the habituation process could also be influenced by emotions and memories. We have not investigated the effect of unpleasant odor on respiratory responses and brain activities, but we hypothesize that at least with a pleasant odor, adaptation decreases the activities of the OFC. A slow and deep respiratory pattern returns to normal breathing. However, with the desensitization to odor, sustained activities in ENT and HI were observed; this might be the remaining activity without feedback from the OFC. What is the role of adaption in olfaction? We suggest that sustained activation in ENT and HI during the adaptation period have a potential to sensitize rapidly impending new events.

Acknowledgements
The authors are grateful to The Cosmetology Research Foundation for their support.

References

Boiten FA, Frijda NH, Wientjes CJE (1994). Emotions and respiratory pattern : Review and critical analysis. International J of Psychophysiol 17: 103-128.
Davis M (1992). The role of the amygdala in fear and anxiety. Ann Rev of Neurosci 15: 353-375.
Ekman G., Berglund B, Berglund U, (1967). Lindvall T. Perceived intensity of odor as a function of time of adaptation. Scand. J. Psychol 8: 177-86.
Homma I, Masaoka Y, Hirasawa K, Yamane F, Hori T (2001) Comparison of source localization of interictal epileptic spike potentials in patients estimated by the dipole tracing method with the focus directly recorded by the depth electrodes. Neurosci Lett 304: 1-4.
Inoue M, Masaoka Y, Kawamura M, Okamoto Y and Homma I (2008) Differences in areas of human frontal medial wall activated by left and right motor execution: Dipole-tracing analysis of grand-averaged potentials incorporated with MNI three-layer head model. Neurosci Lett 437: 82-87.
Kurahashi T, Menini A (1997) Mechanism odorant adaptation in the olfactory receptor cell. Nature 385: 725-729.
Levy LM, Henkin RI, Hutter A, Lin CS, Martins D, Schellinger D (1997) Functional MRI of human olfaction. J Comput Assist Tomogr 21:849-56.
Masaoka Y., Homma I (2004) Amygdala and emotional breathing. In: Champag-

nat J (ed) Post-genomic perspectives in modeling and control of breathing. Kluwer Academic/Plenum Publishers, New York, pp9-14.

Masaoka Y, Koiwa N, Homma I (2005) Inspiratory phase-locked alpha oscillation in human olfaction: source generators estimated by a dipole tracing method. J Physiol 566(3): 979-97.

Masaoka Y, Yoshimura N, Kawamura M, Inoue M, Homma I (2006) Impairment of odor recognition in Parkinson's disease caused by weak activations of the orbitofrotal cortex. Neuroscience Letter 412:45-50.

Okamoto Y, Homma I (2004) Development of a user-friendly EEG analyzing system specialized for the equivalent dipole method Int J Bioelectromagn [serial online; Vol 6: No1] Available at:
http://www.ijbem.org/volume6/number1/005.htm.

Poellinger A, Thomas R, Lio P, Lee A, Makris N, Rosen BR, Kwong KK (2001) Activation and habituation in olfaction –An fMRI study. Neuroimage, 13: 547-560.

Rolls ET (2001) The rules of formation of the olfactory representations found in the orbitofrontal cortex olfactory areas in primates. Chem Senses 26: 595-604.

Royet JP, Zald D, Versace R, Costes N, Lavenne F, Koenig O, Gervais R (2000) Emotional responses to pleasant and unpleasant olfactory, visual, and auditory stimuli: a positron emission tomography study. J Neurosci 20: 7752-59.

Shipley MT, Ennis M (1996) Functional organization of olfactory system. J Neurobiol 30: 123-176.

Sobel N, Prabhakaran V, Desmond JE, Glover GH, Goode RL, Sullivan EV, Gabrieli JDE (1998) Sniffing and smelling: separate subsystems in the human olfactory cortex. Nature 392: 282-286.

Wilson DA (1998) Habituation of odor responses in the rat anterior piriform cortex. J Neurophysiol 79: 1425-1440.

Role of the medial frontal wall for readiness of motor execution

Manabu Inoue [1,2], Yuri Masaoka [1], Mitsuru Kawamura [2], Yoshiwo Okamoto [3], and Ikuo Homma [1]

[1]Department of Physiology, Showa University School of Medicine, 1-5-8 Hatanodai, Shinagawa-ku, Tokyo 142-8555, Japan
<e-mail> gakinoue@med.showa-u.ac.jp
[2]Department of Neurology, Showa University School of Medicine, 1-5-8 Hatanodai, Shinagawa-ku, Tokyo 142-8555, Japan
[3]Department of Electrical, Electronics and Computer Engineering, Faculty of Engineering, Chiba Institute of Technology, 2-17-1 Tsudanuma, Narashino-shi, Chiba 275-0016, Japan

Summary. The sensorimotor area and supplementary motor area and cingulate cortex of the frontal medial wall are reported to be important for the generation and control of movements, according to neuroimaging studies and electroencephalography (EEG) recordings with subdural electrodes. Combining these advantages of EEG with dipole-tracing analysis incorporating a realistic three-layer head model (scalp-skull-brain head model; SSB/DT) allows for the detection of dipoles in the millisecond range and investigation of the processing of cognitive function and movement execution. In this study, we constructed a scalp-skull-brain head model from Montreal Neurological Institute standard brain images and detected dipole localizations in the millisecond range from grand-averaged negative slope (NS) to motor potentials during a simple pinching movement. The simple self-initiated left and right motor execution activated different areas: the left movement activated the presupplementary motor area (pre-SMA), putamen, rostral cingulate cortex and rostral premotor area, which are associated with cognitive functions and self-initiated decisions. These areas were associated with the early NS potential during left pinching movement preparation. The right movement activated the caudal cingulate cortex, pre-SMA and caudal premotor area, and these areas were activated just before the execution of movement.

In the primary stage of the cognitive circuit for motor control, pre-SMA-putamen are activated before the onset of NS that relates cognitive function as decision making, response selection in time perception and motivation.

Key words. EEG, dipole-tracing analysis, MNI, pre-SMA, putamen

Introduction

Movement-related cortical potentials (MRCPs) can be recorded from scalp electrodes and precede and follow voluntary movements (Kornhuber and Deecke 1965; Shibasaki et al. 1980; Barret et al. 1986). MRCPs are composed of three waveforms observed in the averaged electroencephalogram: the readiness potential, originally termed the Bereitschafts potential (BP), the negative slope (NS) and the motor potential (MP). The BP is a slow negative potential that occurs 1-2 s before a self-paced voluntary movement (Kornhuber and Deeke 1965). The NS is a negative potential that occurs 200-500 ms before the onset of electromyography (EMG) activity. (Shibasaki et al. 1980), and the MP occurs approximately 100 ms after, or occasionally before, EMG onset.

Functional magnetic resonance imaging (fMRI) and positron emission tomography (PET) have reported the areas related to MRCPs (Rao et al. 1993; Toma et al. 1999; Cunnington et al. 2002; Shibasaki et al. 1993). These studies showed that the contralateral sensorimotor area (SM1) and bilateral supplementary motor area (SMA) are consistently activated in association with finger movement. Studies with high temporal-resolution electroencephalography (EEG) recording with subdural electrodes have shown that the SMA plays important roles in unilateral and bilateral movements, whereas the primary motor area is involved in the preparation of contralateral movements (Ikeda et al. 1995).

The SMA is categorized into the pre-SMA, which projects to primary motor cortex areas involved in higher-order functions such as planning (He et al. 1995; Wang et al. 2001), and the SMA proper which has direct spinal projections and is involved in movement (Lu et al. 1994). Both the pre-SMA and SMA proper are involved in self-generated movements. Although neuroimaging and EEG studies have shown areas related to MRCPs, it is not yet incomplete to detect areas involved in MRCP processing.

EEG is a non-invasive technique for monitoring brain electrical activity and has good time resolution. Combining these advantages of EEG with the dipole-tracing analysis incorporating a realistic three-layer head model ; (SSB/DT) (Homma et al. 1994, 1995) allows for the detection of dipoles in the ms range. The reliability of source localization from field potentials has been tested in patients with focal epileptic seizures undergoing presurgical evaluation with intracranial subdural strip electrodes (Homma et al. 1994) and with depth electrodes (Homma et al. 2001). SSB/DT has been used to localize source generators of MRCPs (Kanamaru et al. 1999) and in the analyses recognition for facial expression in patients with Parkinson disease (Yoshimura et al. 2005) and in the analysis of olfaction (Masaoka et al. 2005). SSB/DT allows for the estimation of dipole locations in deep structures of the brain such as the amygdala, entorhinal cortex, hippocampus and orbitofrontal cortex.

SSB/DT can be used for functional brain mapping in humans; however, it may be difficult to perform dipole analysis in routine experiments or clinical examinations. This method uses a realistic three-dimensional head model of MR images from each subject segmented into brain, skull and scalp aspects. However, MR images are not always available and can be expensive. To address these issues, dipole analysis has been performed with a spherical three-shell model (Tarkka and Treede 1993) for source localization of pain-related somatosensory evoked potentials, and obtained dipole locations are superimposed on a standard brain MR image (Shimojo et al. 2000). Silva et al. (1999) reported that dipole locations incorporated onto a standard realistic model are useful in the event that imaging is not available.

The Montreal Neurological Institute (MNI) standard coordinate system is the most commonly used streotaxic platform (Brett et al. 2002). A standard MNI template was created from MR images from 152 subjects, and neuroimaging data were used to create normalized MNI brain coordinates associated with Talairach brain coordinates (Collins et al. 1994). The MNI coordinate uses three-dimensional signal-source estimation algorithms such as low-resolution brain electromagnetic tomography (LORETA) for EEG (Pascual-Marqui et al. 2002) and Near-Infrared Spectroscopy (NIRS) (Okamoto and Homma 2004; Singh et al. 2005).

In this study, we constructed a scalp-skull-brain head model from the standard MNI brain images and detected dipole localizations from grand-averaged NS to MP in the millisecond range.

Materials and methods

Three subjects were healthy volunteers (all men; age 30, 34 and 55 years). All subjects were right-handed as confirmed by the Edinburgh Handedness Inventory (Oldfield 1971). Informed consent was obtained from each subject, and the study confirmed to the guidelines of the Ethics Committee of the Showa University School of Medicine. The subjects were instructed to perform a self-paced pinching movement with the index finger and thumb of the right or left hand approximately every 20 s. Right and left pinching movements were performed separately, approximately 100 times each. The subjects were instructed to avoid other movements, and eyes were closed.

Electroencephalograms were obtained with 19 Ag/AgCl electrodes attached to the scalp according to the international 10-20 system with a reference electrode attached to the right earlobe. Electrode impedances were maintained at less than 5 Ω throughout the recordings. Potentials were amplified and band-pass filtered (0.03-100.00 Hz) by the EEG recorder (EEG-1100; Nihon Kohden, Tokyo Japan), and data were stored on an EEG analyzer (DAE-2100; Nihon Kohden). The data were sampled at 1-ms intervals and stored on magnetic optical disks for off-line analysis. Electro-oculograms were recorded with electrodes placed at the inferior lateral canthus and supraorbital to the right eye. The surface EMG activity of the left and right abductor pollicis brevis muscles was recorded with an amplifier (AB-621G; Nihon Kohden). The onset of EMG activity was used to average signals from all subjects ranging from 1500 ms before EMG activity to 100 ms after EMG activity. For the off-line analysis of the data, waveforms were eliminated for trials compromised by blinking or excessive eye or body movements (>20 µV). Trails associated with a steep EMG wave or eye movement, body movement, or an artifact 2 s before to 1 s after EMG onset were also eliminated.

MRCPs averaged within subject were analyzed with an SSB/DT incorporating the subject's head model, and grand-averaged MRCPs across the subjects were analyzed with an SSB/DT incorporating the MNI three-layer head model. A detailed description of the SSB/DT method has been reported elsewhere. SSB/DT involves calculation of the location of source generators in the brain from the electroencephalographic data. The actual potential field distribution recorded from the 19 scalp electrodes (V_{meas}) was compared with the calculated field distribution (V_{cal}) for an appropriately equivalent current dipole (for one-dipole estimations) or two appropriately equivalent dipoles (for two-dipole estimations). The inverse solution (He et al. 1987) was used to determine the dipole location and orientation that best fitted the recorded data. The locations and vector moments of one- or two- current dipoles were iteratively changed within the head model until the minimal squared difference between V_{meas} and V_{cal} was obtained by the simplex method (Kowalik et al. 1968). The degree of source concentration can be calculated in terms of dipolarity (D[%]). A dipolarity of 100% is ideal; however, in practice it is usually less than 100% due to noise, electrode misalignment or non-dipole components of the electric sources. In the present study, dipolarity greater than 98% was considered to indicate a concentrated source (Homma et al., 2004). Conductivities of the brain (0.33 S/m), skull (0.0041 S/m) and scalp (0.33 S/m) were incorporated into the calculation. The unconstrained one-moving-dipole model was used in the present study.

The onset of the BP and the peak latencies of NS and MP for each subject were measured as averaged individual waveforms. Differences between right and left BP, NS and MP latencies were compared by Wilcoxson's signed-rank test. Root mean square (RMS) values of the MP were measured with the SSB/DT software (BS-navi), and differences between right and left RMS values of the MP were compared with Wilcoxson's signed-rank test. Activated areas were indicated by a dipolarity (goodness-of-fit) of greater than 98% and were computed automatically in MNI brain coordinates.

Results

BP, NS or MP latencies did not differ significantly between the left and right pinching movements (BP, P=0.93, NS, P=1, MP, P=0.66) (Table 1). The RMS value for MP did not differ significantly between the left and right movements (P=0.43) (Table 2). Grand-averaged data across the subjects is shown in Fig.1. RMS values and goodness-of-fit (%) dipolarity; are shown below the grand-averaged MRCPs. RMS values increased from NS to MP.

Dipole localizations over ~50 ms from NS to MP are shown in Fig.2.and 3. Dipoles converged in specific areas related to motor activity. During the left pinching movements (Fig.2), from -250 ms to -100 ms, dipoles were detected in the right pre-SMA (BA 6) and the rostral cingulate (BA 24). From -100 ms to -50 ms, these dipoles were constantly detected in right cingulate gyrus. At -50 ms, the dipoles moved to the right lateral premotor cortex, and at the onset of movement, the dipoles converged in the right motor area.

Right pinching movement dipoles converged in more specific areas than those of the left pinching movement (Fig.3). During the late component of

Table 1. BP, NS or MP latencies between the left and right pinching movements

Latency (ms)	Left	Right
BP	−1202 ± 60 *	−1208 ± 85 *
NS	− 435 ± 86 **	−435 ± 124 **
MP	196 ± 52 ***	193 ± 31 ***

* P=0.93; ** P=1; *** P=0.66 vs. left and right
BP, bereitschafts potential; NS, negative slope; MP, motor potential. Modified from Neuroscience Letter 2008, Inoue et al.

Table 2. RMS value for MP between the left and right movements

RMS (μ V)	Left	Right
MP	1.65 ± 0.69	1.38 ± 0.60

P=0.43 vs. left and right
RMS, root mean square. Modified from Neuroscience Letter 2008, Inoue et al.

NS from -250 ms to -50 ms, dipoles converged in the left caudal cingulate area (BA 24). Dipoles in the left caudal cingulate area remained until 50 ms before movement onset. At 50 ms before movement onset, dipoles moved to the left pre-SMA and the left premotor cortex. At movement onset, dipoles were detected in the left motor area.

Also Fig 2 and 3 lists the MNI coordinates of dipole localizations shown, and brain regions were confirmed by the atlas of Talairach and Tournoux (Talairach and Tournoux 1988).

Discussion

Dipole estimation from grand-averaged data incorporating the MNI three-layer head model

We performed dipole estimation from grand-averaged NS to MP potentials during voluntary pinching movement; this estimation incorporated the MNI three-layer head model. The measured data may include environmental noise and background activity, resulting in scattered dipole localization. The advantage of group-averaged data is that the signal-to-noise ratio can be enhanced by averaging. If the stimuli are well controlled, individual averaged potentials can include similar components across subjects, and similar dipole traces can be obtained over time. Dipole estimation from group-averaged data can be applied to a normalized gross brain. Thus, the MNI model is suitable for dipole estimation with group-averaged data. The positions of the 10-20 standard electrodes were adequately cast on the

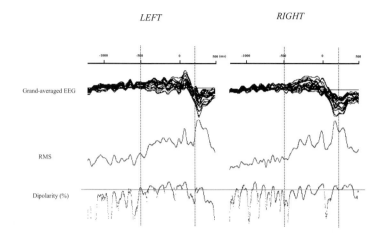

Fig.1. Grand-averaged data across the subjects is shown. RMS values and goodness-of-fit (%) dipolarity; are shown below the grand-averaged MRCPs. RMS values increased from NS to MP. Modified from Neuroscience Letter 2008, Inoue et al. Refer to color plates

MNI head model and were based on anatomic landmarks that could be normalized to standard streotaxic coordinates. Okamoto et al. (Okamoto et al 2004) reported NIRS imaging data utilizing an MNI three-dimensional anatomic platform to provide anatomic information.

A previous study using a standard realistic head model for EEG source reconstruction indicated that a standardized realistic head model performs better than a spherical model (Fuchs et al. 2002). Verkindt et al. (1995) reported no significant differences in dipole locations between individual and grand-averaged data sets. However, Whittingstall et al. (2003) reported average differences in dipole locations between individual and group-averaged data sets of approximately 1.1 cm. In the present study, we found dipoles in specific anatomic regions related to NS to MP potentials, and the coordinates were confirmed by the atlas of Talairach and Tournoux (Talairach and Tournoux 1988). Thus, group-averaged data sets obtained with a standard averaged brain model are valid for detecting typical localizations. In addition, averaged data can be used to detect dipole movements in the ms range.

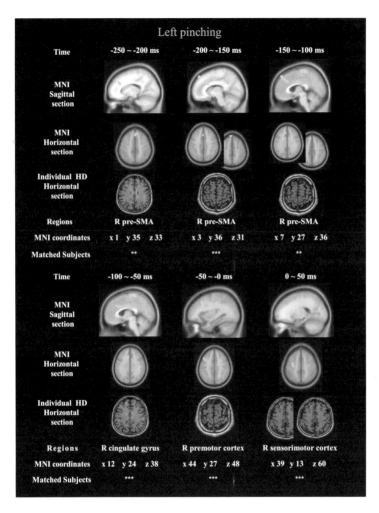

Fig.2. Dipole estimation of ground averaged MRCP of all the subjects incorporate with MNI standard brain by left pinching movements and typical example of dipole localization estimated from MRCP of single subject incorporate with individual head model. Regions in brain are also shown and the * stands for subjects' numbers whose dipoles appeared in each regions. Dipoles greater than 98 % were indicated pre 250 to post 50 ms in order of 50 ms. Modified from Neuroscience Letter 2008, Inoue et al. Refer to color plates

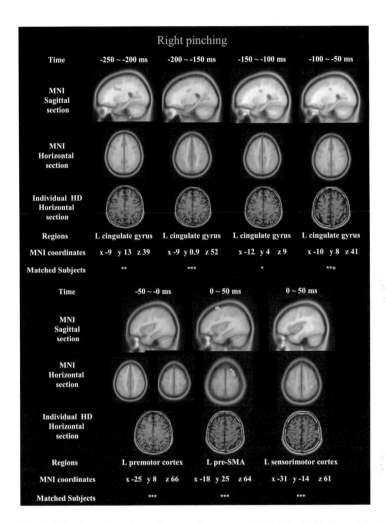

Fig.3. Dipole estimation of ground averaged MRCP of all the subjects incorporate with MNI standard brain by right pinching movements and typical example of dipole localization estimated from MRCP of single subject incorporate with individual head model. Regions in brain are also shown and the * stands for subjects' numbers whose dipoles appeared in each regions. Dipoles greater than 98 % were indicated pre 250 to post 50 ms in order of 50 ms. Modified from Neuroscience Letter 2008, Inoue et al. Refer to color plates

Processing of motor activation

Results of the present study confirmed that the generators for the NS potential are localized in the contralateral pre-SMA, cingulate motor area and lateral prefrontal area. During the MP potential, dipoles converged in the contralateral sensorimotor hand area. These results were consistent with those of previous studies (Shibasaki et al. 1980, 1993; Neshige et al. 1988; Rao et al, 1993; Toma et al. 1999; Cunnington et al. 2002). The time resolution of dipole analysis allowed us to detect dipoles in the ms range from the NS to the MP. Subjects performed simple self-paced pinching movements; however, we found a difference in motor area of activation between the left and right pinching movements, and we also found that the appearance of dipoles in these motor-related areas converged at different times between the left and right movements. Large differences between the left and right pinching movement were identified in areas of activations. pre-SMA, caudate nucleus, putamen and pre-motor area were activated during the early onset of the NS potential in the left pinching movement, and activation of anterior cingulate motor areas for left movement and the posterior cingulate for right movement.

Activations of the media frontal wall

A number of studies have shown involvement of the frontal medial wall in the generation and control movement (Picard and Strick 2001; Cunnington et al. 2002). The medial wall contains three motor areas: the SMA proper, the pre-SMA and the cingulate motor area. The SMA proper, located in the caudal portion of area 6, projects directly to the primary motor areas and to the spinal cords (He et al. 1995). The pre-SMA, located to the rostral portion of premotor areas is interconnected with the prefrontal cortex. These differences in connectivity are reflected in the different pattern of activation in these two supplementary motor areas. The SMA proper is predominantly involved in direct motor execution, whereas, the pre-SMA is concerned with cognitive and sensory inputs for motor control. SMA proper activation is related to simple tasks, the activations simply related to the motor execution (Hikosaka et al. 1996), whereas, and activation of the pre-SMA occurs in parallel with the acquisition of motor-sequence tasks. The pre-SMA is activated when the movement is more complex and requires visual or auditory motor association and learning. The pre-SMA is also involved in self-generated tasks (Deiber et al. 1999) and is activated in early movement preparation (Lee et al. 1999). In the present study, activation of the pre-SMA was observed during the early onset of the NS in the left self-initiated movement, indicating that cognitive or attentional aspects of motor control are necessary for left hand execution in the right handed subjects. In addition to the early pre-SMA activation, it was remarkable to observe input from the left pre-SMA to the left putamen during this period.

The SMA projects to the basal ganglia, particularly to the putamen (Takada et al. 1998), and the SMA receives major outputs from the putamen. The basal ganglia and the SMA are involved in perceptual timing tasks as well as motor tasks (Macar et al. 2002), and Ferrandez et al. (2003) suggested that activation of the SMA and left putamen are specific to duration processing. In the first stage of cognitive processing for motor control, the pre-SMA-putamen activates during the early onset of the NS, indicating self initiated left pinching movement may be related more to cognitive functions such as decision making, response selection during time perception and motivation. Activation of these areas was not observed from -500 ms to -300 ms in the right movement execution, but immediately before movement onset at -50 ms, the pre-SMA and pre-motor area were activated. All subjects were right handed in this study, and self- initiated left pinching movements may require more preparation and time-keeping factors for motor execution.

Differences in the activation of cingulate motor area between the left and the right pinching movement

The present study both the left and right pinching movements activated the cingulate motor area, but the left movement activated the anterior portion of the cingulate motor area, and the right movement involved the posterior cingulate motor area. According to Picard and Strick (Picard and Strick 1996), the cingulate motor areas is divided into a rostral cingulate zone with two subdivisions (anterior and posterior) and a caudal cingulate zone. Activation of the anterior cingulate during the left pinching movement corresponded to the posterior rostral cingulate subdivision, and activation of the posterior cingulate corresponded to the caudal cingulated zone. The functions of these areas remain uncertain; however, a recent study reported that the rostral cingulate zone (posterior) is activated during word generation tasks (Crosson et al. 1999) and in tasks involving response selection such as Go/No-Go tasks (Rubia et al. 2001). The rostral cingulate zone (anterior part) is activated to a high degree in response to conflicting or contradictory signals. These tasks require visual motor association, and attentional and cognitive factors. The caudal cingulate zone is activated in association with movement execution (Picard and Strick 1996; Kwan et al. 2000) and is activated along with the SMA proper. Picard and Strick

(Picard and Strick 2001) suggested that the rostral cingulate zone (anterior and posterior) appear to be activated in response to selection and conflict monitoring, and the caudal cingulate zone appears to be activated during simple motor tasks. This functional difference is similar to the differences between the pre-SMA and the SMA proper.

The pre-SMA and the rostral cingulate motor area are activated during internally generated movement (Deiber et al. 1999) and in the early process of movement preparation (Ball et al. 1999). Cunnington et al. (Cunnington et al 2002) reported that the pre-SMA and the rostral cingulated areas appear to be activated during internal preparation and complex movements. They also observed activation of the basal ganglia, in association with internal control and planning. We observed simple self-initiated pinching movements and found that the left pinching movement required more preparation, perceptual timing and motivation, all of which are associated with pre-SMA, putamen (basal ganglia) and the posterior rostral cingulated zone (Inoue et al. 2008). These areas are activated during the early onset of NS. Dipoles in the left caudal cingulate zone remained stable from -350 ms to -50 ms during right pinching movement, and the dipole moved to the left premotor area immediately before movement execution.

The right- hand movement in right-handed subjects requires less activation of those areas activated during the left-hand movement, likely because of the functional plasticity occurs during accustomed movements.

Activation of the premotor cortex before movement execution

Activation of the contralateral premotor cortex is commonly observed just before the onset of movement. However, activation of the premotor cortex during left movement occurs more rostral to activation during right movement. In monkey, the lateral premotor cortex is divided into rostral and caudal divisions (Barbas and Pardya 1987) and the former is commonly associated with the pre-SMA, which is interconnected with the prefrontal cortex, and the latter is a same function as the SMA proper, which projects to the primary motor cortex and the to spinal cord. The pre-SMA and the rostral premotor cortex are more involved in cognitive processing than in motor execution. Again, these differences in the rostral and caudal portions of the premotor cortex could be due to differences in pre-SMA and SMA proper and the rostral and caudal cingulate motor areas with respect to whether they are involved in aspects of cognitive processing or in aspects of motor generation.

The rostral premotor division does not project to the primary motor areas. During the left pinching movement, dipoles in the right rostral premotor area moved directly to the right M1 area. It is possible that the caudal premotor areas are co activated during this period; however, in the present study, we performed one-dipole analysis in which the dipole was estimated in the area generating the strongest currency of polarity. In addition, the lack of dipole convergence in the SMA proper may be due to the fact that strong current polarity in area M1 is drawn toward area M1 rather than SMA proper; the SMA proper is directly connected to area M1, and is involved in motor generation. Motor areas of the medial wall discussed above may be activated in parallel, and in this case, dipoles could be scattered in two-dipole analysis. There are limitations of single- dipole analysis. However, we able to detect areas generating strong polarization in the ms range and clearly identified functional differences in each area.

In summary, even in simple self-initiated motor tasks, left and right motor executions activate different areas; the former activates the pre-SMA, putamen, rostral cingulate cortex and rostral premotor areas, which are associated with cognitive processing and self-initiated decisions. These areas were activated during early processing in left pinching movement preparation. The latter activates the caudal cingulate cortex, pre-SMA and caudal premotor area, which were activated just before movement execution. The temporal resolution of dipole detection shown in the present study can applied to the analysis of the motor processing in patients with injury to the motor areas and in patients with movement disorders such as Parkinson disease.

References

Ball, T., Schreiber, A., Feige, B., Wagner, M., Lucking, C.H., Kristeva-Feige, R., 1999. The role of higher-order motors area in voluntary movement as revealed by high-resolution EEG and fMRI. Neuroimage 10, 682–694.

Barbas, H., Pandya, D.N., 1987. Architecture and frontal cortical connections of the premotor cortex (area 6) in the rhesus monkey. J. Comp. Neurol. 256, 211–228.

Barrett, G., Shibasaki, H., Negishe, R, 1986. Cortical potentials preceding voluntary movement: evidence for three periods of preparation in man. Electroencephalogr. Clin. Neurophysiol. 63, 327–339.

Brett, M., Johnsrude, I.S., Owen, A.M. 2002. The problem of functional localization in the human brain. Nat. Rev. Neurosci. 3, 243–249.

Collins, D.L., Neelin, P., Peters, T.M., Evans, A.C., 1994. Automatic 3D intersubject registration of MR volumetric data in standardized Talairach space. J. Comput. Assist. Tomogr. 18, 192–205.

Crosson, B., Sadek, J.R., Bobholz, J.A., Gokcay, D., Mohr, C.M., Leonard, C.M., Maron, L., Auerbach, E.J., Browd, S.R., Freeman, A.J., Briggs, R.W., 1999.

Activity in the paracingulate and cingulate sulci during word generation: an fMRI study of functional anatomy. Cereb. Cortex 9, 307—316.

Cunnington, R., Windischberger, C., Deecke, L., Moser, E., 2002. The preparation and execution of self-initiated and externally-triggered movement: a study of event-related fMRI. Neuroimage 15, 373—385.

Deiber, M. P., Honda, M., Ibanez, V., Sadato, N., Hallett, M., 1999. Mesial motor areas in self-initiated versus externally triggered movements examined with fMRI: effect of movement type and rate. J. Neurophysiol. 81, 3065—3077.

Ferrandez, A.M., Hugueville, L., Lehericy, S., Poline, J.B., Marsault, C., Pouthas, V., 2003. Basal ganglia and supplementary motor area subtend duration perception: an fMRI study. Neuroimage 19, 1532—1544.

Fuchs, M., Kastner, J., Wagner, M., Hawes, S., Ebersole, J.S., 2002. A standardized boundary element method volume conductor model. Clin. Neurophysiol. 113, 702—12.

He, B., Musha, T., Okamoto, Y., Homma, S., Nakajima, Y., Sato, T., 1987. Electric dipole tracing in the brain by means of the boundary element method and its accuracy. IEEE Trans. Biomed. Eng. 34, 406—14.

He, S.Q., Dum, R.P., Strick, P.L., 1995. Topographic organization of corticospinal projections from the frontal lobe: motor areas on the medial surface of the hemisphere. J. Neurosci. 15, 3284—3306.

Hikosaka, O., Sakai, K., Miyauchi, S., Takino, R., Sasaki, Y., Putz, B. 1996. Activation of human presupplimentary motor area in learning of sequential procedures: a functional MRI study. J. Neurophysiol. 76, 617—621.

Homma, S., Musha, T., Nakajima, Y., Okamoto, Y., Blom, S., Flink, R., Hagbarth, K.E., Mustrom, U., 1994. Location of electric current sources in the human brain estimated by the dipole tracing method of the scalp-skull-brain (SSB) head model. Electroencephalogr. Clin. Neurophysiol. 91, 374—382.

Homma, S., Musha, T., Nakajima, Y., Okamoto, Y., Blom, S., Flink, R., Hagbarth, K.E., 1995. Conductivity ratios of the scalp-skull-brain head model in estimating equivalent dipole sources in human brain. Neurosci. Res. 22, 51—5.

Homma, I., Masaoka, Y., Hirasawa, K., Yamane, F., Hori, T., Okamoto, Y., 2001. Comparison of source localization of interictal epileptic spike potentials in patients estimated by the dipole tracing method with the focus directly recorded by the depth electrodes. Neurosci. Lett. 304, 1—4.

Ikeda, A., Luders, H.O., Shibasaki, H., Collura, T.F., Burgess, R.C., Morris, H.H.3rd., Hamano., T. 1995. Movement-related potentials associated with bilateral simultaneous and unilateral movements recorded from human supplementary motor area. Electroencephalogr. Clin. Neurophysiol. 95, 323—334.

Inoue M, Masaoka Y, Kawamura M, Okamoto Y, Homma I 2008 Differences in areas of human frontal medial wall activated by left and right motor execution: Dipole-tracing analysis of grand-averaged potentials incorporated with MNI three-layer head model. Neuroscience Letters, 437, 82-87

Kanamaru, A., Homma, I., Hara, T., 1999. Movement related cortical source for elbow flexion in patients with brachial plexus injury after intercostal-musculocutaneous nerve crossing. Neurosci. Lett. 274, 203—206.

Kornhuber, H.H., Deecke, L. 1965. Changes in the brain potential in voluntary

movements and passive movements in man: readiness potential and reafferent potentials. Pflugers Archiv. Gesamte Physiol. Menscheu. Tieve 284, 1—17.
Kowalik, J., Osborn, M.R. 1968. Methods for unconstrained optimization problems. American Elsevier Publishing, New York.
Kwan, C.L., Crawley, A.P., Mikulis, D.J., Davis, K.D., 2000. An fMRI study of the anterior cingulate cortex and surrounding medial wall activations evoked by noxious cutaneous heat and cold stimuli. Pain 85, 359—374.
Lee, K.M., Chang, K.H., Roh, J.K., 1999. Subregions within the supplementary motor area activated at different stages of movement preparation and execution. Neuroimage 9, 117—123.
Lu, M.T., Preston, J.B., Strick, P.L., 1994. Interconnections between the prefrontal cortex and the premotor areas in the frontal lobe. J. Comp. Neurol. 341, 375—392.
Macar, F., Lejeune, H., Bonnet, M., Ferrara, M., Pouthas, V., Vidal, F., Maquet, P. 2002. Activation of the supplementary motor area and of attentional networks during temporal processing. Exp. Brain Res. 142, 475—485.
Masaoka, Y., Koiwa, N., Homma, I. 2005. Inspiratory phase-locked alpha oscillationin human olfaction: source generators estimated by a dipole tracing method. J. Physiol.566, 979—97.
Neshige, R., Luders, H., Shibasaki, H., 1988. Recording of movement-related potentials from scalp and cortex in man. Brain 111, 719—736.
Okamoto, M., Dan, H., Sakamoto, K., Takeo, K., Shimizu, K., Kohno, S., Oda, I., Isobe, S., Suzuki, T., Kohyama, K., Dan, I., 2004. Three-dimensional probabilistic anatomical cranio-cerebral correlation via the international 10-20 system oriented for transcranial functional brain mapping. Neuroimage 21, 99—111.
Okamoto, Y., Homma, I., 2004. Development of a user-friendly EEG analyzing system specialized for the equivalent dipole method. Int. J. Bioelectromagn. [serial online; Vol 6: No1] Available at: http://www.ijbem.org/volume6/number1/005.htm.
Oldfield, R.C., 1971. The assessment and analysis of handedness: the Edinburah inventory. Neuropsychologia. 9, 97—113.
Pascual-Marqui, R.D., Esslen, M., Kochi, K., Lehmann, D., 2002. Functional imaging with low-resolution brain electromagnetic tomography (LORETA): a review. Methods Find. Exp. Clin. Pharmacol. 24, 91—95.
Picard, N., Strick, P.L., 1996. Motor areas of the medial wall: a review of their location and functional activation. Cereb. Cortex 6, 342—353.
Picard, N., Strick, P.L., 2001. Imaging the premotor areas. Curr. Opin. Neurobiol. 11, 663—672.
Rao, S.M., Binder, J.R., Bandettini, P.A., Hammeke, T.A., Yetkin, F.Z., Jesmanowicz, A., Lisk, L.M., Morris, G.L., Muller, W.M., Estkowski, L.D. 1993. Functional magnetic resonance imaging of complex human movements. Neurology 43, 2311—2318.
Rubia, K., Russell, T., Overmeyer, S., brammer, M.J., Bullmore, E.T., Sharma, T., Simmons, A., Williams, S.C., Giampietro, V., Andrew, C.M., Taylor, E., 2001. Mapping motor inhibition: conjunctive brain activations across different ver-

sions of go/no-go and stop tasks. Neuroimage 13, 250—261.
Shibasaki, H., Barrett, G., Halliday, E., Halliday, A.M., 1980. Components of the movement-related cortical potential and their scalp topography. Electroencephalogr. Clin. Neurophysiol. 49, 213—226.
Shibasaki, H., Sadato, N. Lyshkow, H., Yonekura, Y., Honda, M., Nagamine, T., Suwazono, S., Magata, Y., Ikeda, A., Miyazaki, M. et al., 1993. Both primary motor cortex and supplementary motor area play an important role in complex finger movement. Brain. 116, 1387—1398.
Shimojo, M., svensson, P., Arendt-Nielsen, L., Chen, A.C., 2000. Dynamic brain topography of somatosensory evoked potentials and equivalent dipoles in response to graded painful skin and muscle stimulation. Brain Topogr. 13, 43—58.
Silva, C., Almeida, R., Oostendorp, T., Ducla-Soares, E., Foreid, J.P., Pimentel, T., 1999. Interictal spike localization using a standard realistic head model: simulations and analysis of clinical data. Clin. Neurophysiol. 110, 846—855.
Singh, A.K., Okamoto, M., Dan, H., Jurcak, V., Dan, I., 2005. Spatial r egistration of multichannel multi-subject fNIRS data to MNI space without MRI. Neuroimage 27, 842—851.
Takada, M., Tokuno, H., Nambu, A., Inase, M., 1998. Corticostriatal projections from the somatic motor areas of the frontal cortex in the macaque monkey: segregation versus overlap of input zones from the primary motor cortex, the supplementary motor area, and the premotor cortex. Exp. Brain. Res. 120, 114—128.
Talairach, J., Tournoux, P., 1988. Co-Planar Stereotaxic Atlas of the Human Brain:3-Dimentional Proportional System: An Approach to Cerebral Imaging. Thieme Med. Pub., Stuttgart.
Tarkka, I.M., Treede, R.D., 1993. Equivalent electrical source analysis of pain-related somatosensory evoked potentials elicited by a CO2 laser. J. Clin. Neurophysiol. 10, 513—519.
Toma, K., Honda, M., Hanakawa, T., Okada, t., Fukuyama, H., Ikeda, A., Nishizawa, S., Konishi, J., Shibasaki, H., 1999. Activities of the primary and supplementary motor areas increase in preparation and execution of voluntary muscle relaxation: an event-related fMRI study. J. Neurosci. 19, 3527—3534.
Verkindt, C., Bertrand, O., Perrin, F., Echallier, J.F., Pernier, J., 1995. Tonotopic organization of the human auditory cortex N100 topography and multiple dipole model analysis. J. Electroencephalogr. Clin. Neurophysiol. 96, 143—156.
Wang, Y., Shima, K., Sawamura, H., Tanji, J., 2001. Spatial distribution of cingulate cells projecting to the primary, supplementary, and presupplementary motor areas: a retrograde multiple labeling study in the macaque monkey. Neurosci. Res. 39, 39—49.
Whittingstall, K., Stroink, G., Gates, L., Connolly, J.F, Finley, A., 2003. Effects of dipole position, orientation and noise on the accuracy of EEG source localization. Biomed. Eng. Online 2, 14.
Yoshimura, N., Kawamura, M., Masaoka, Y., Homma, I. 2005. The amygdala of patients with Parkinson's disease is silent in response to fearful facial expressions. Neuroscience 131: 523-34.

Poster Presentations

Ryanodine receptor type 1 / calcium release channel in the endoplasmic reticulum as the target of nitric oxide to cause the intracellular calcium signaling

Hideto Oyamada[1], Toshiko Yamazawa[2], Takashi Murayama[3], Takahiro Hayashi[1], Takashi Sakurai[3], Masamitsu Iino[2] and Katsuji Oguchi[1]

[1]Department of Pharmacology, Showa University School of Medicine, 1-5-8 Hatanodai, Shinagawa-ku, Tokyo 142-8555, Japan
[2]Department of Molecular Cellular Pharmacology, University of Tokyo Graduated School of Medicine, 7-3-1 Hongo, Bunkyo-ku, Tokyo 113-0033
[3]Deparment of Pharmacology, Juntendo University School of Medicine, 2-1-1 Hongo, Bunkyo-ku, Tokyo 113-8421 Japan

Summary. Ryanodine receptors (RyRs) are the calcium (Ca^{2+}) release channels that are mainly distributed in excitable cells containing neuronal cells. The type 1 of RyR isoforms (RyR1) is highly expressed in the Purkinje cells (PCs) of the cerebellum. Recently the synaptic nitric oxide (NO) signals were detected from the parallel fiber (PF) to PCs dependent on the frequency of PF activity that induced the long-term potentiation. To examine whether or not the NO can activate the RyR1 to increase the intracellular Ca^{2+} concentration ($[Ca^{2+}]_i$), we have employed the inducible recombinant RyR1 expression system of HEK293 cell and its $[Ca^{2+}]_i$ imaging. NOC7, a NO donor, could cause dose-dependent increases in the $[Ca^{2+}]_i$ in the wild - type RyR1 expressing cells but not in the S - nitrosation site - deficient RyR1 mutant expressing cells. The increments of $[Ca^{2+}]_i$ elicited by NOC7 were inhibited by the pretreatment of ryanodine, a open-locked channel blocker of RyRs, but not by ODQ, a soluble guanylate cyclase inhibitor. These results suggest that the NO can evoked intracellular Ca^{2+} signals resulted from the Ca^{2+} release through the RyR1 activation by the S - nitrosation.

Key Words. Ryanodine receptor, Calcium, Nitric oxide

1 Introduction

Calcium (Ca^{2+}) is one of the most ubiquitous intracellular second messengers and is responsible for various important cell functions. In nerve cells, changes in intracellular Ca^{2+} concentrations ($[Ca^{2+}]_i$) have been reported to regulate excitability, neurotransmitter release, metabolic reaction and gene expression (Berridge 1998). In response to the various signals, the $[Ca^{2+}]_i$ can rise as results from the extracellular Ca^{2+} influx through the plasma membrane cation channels and /or the intracellular Ca^{2+} release from the endoplasmic reticulum though the Ca^{2+} release channels. Ryanodine receptors (RyRs) are one of the Ca^{2+} release channel families and mainly distributed in excitable cells to function as the Ca^{2+} - induced Ca^{2+} release channels, which are thought to be able to amplify the local elementary Ca^{2+} signals into the global Ca^{2+} waves or Ca^{2+} oscillations in a single cell.

Nitric oxide (NO) is also an intracellular messenger, the role of which was first recognized as the endothelium - derived relaxing factor (EDRF) and one subtype of NO synthases have been identified mainly in the nervous system called neuronal NOS (nNOS) (Zhang and Snyder 1995). In the cerebellum, for example, nNOS is expressed in granule cells but not Purkinje Cells (PCs) (Bredt et al. 1990) and the long – term potentiation (LTP) at the parallel fiber (PF) - PC synapse is NO dependent because it is blocked by a NOS inhibitor and a NO donor application induces LTP in slice preparations (Lev-Ram et al. 2002). Furthermore, PF stimulation – induced NO signals within PCs were detected and the NO release levels from the PF terminals had the same biphasic dependence on the frequency of PF stimulations as the LTP generation at the PF-PC synapse had. (Namiki et al. 2005). Thus, NO is now considered to be produced by firing neurons and spread over synaptic clefts to reach postsynaptic cells, contributing to the various neuronal functions including synaptic plasticity (Iino 2006).

Signaling downstream of NO has been characterized at first pharmacologically to confirm its activation of soluble guanylate cyclase (sGC) to produce cyclic GMP (cGMP) and subsequent stimulation of cGMP - dependent protein kinase (PKG) (Ignarro and Kadowitz 1985). But other molecules as the physiological target of NO in PC are proposed including divers range of effects on metalloproteins, enzymes, cation channels, transcription factors, nucleic acids and lipids (Edwards and Rickard 2007). In this study, we focused on the possibility of the RyR / calcium release channel as the target molecules of NO to cause the intracellular Ca^{2+} signaling.

2 Experimental models and Results

In PCs of cerebellum previously described, the type 1 RyR (RyR1) is highly expressed between three RyR isoforms identified in vertebrates (Furuichi et al. 1994). Therefore, we employed a stable line of HEK293 cells with tetracycline - inducible expression of exogenous RyR1 and analyzed the effects of NOC7, a NO donor, on the $[Ca^{2+}]_i$ in these cells with a fluorescent Ca^{2+} indicator Fura2.

The application of NOC7 increased $[Ca^{2+}]_i$ in HEK293 cells expressing exogenous RyR1 but not in non - induced HEK293 cells, which did not express exogenous RyR1. The transient increase in $[Ca^{2+}]_i$ could be observed even in the absence of extracellular Ca^{2+}, suggesting that NOC7 - induced Ca^{2+} increases were results from the release of Ca^{2+} stored in the intracellular Ca^{2+} store sites. (Fig. 1)

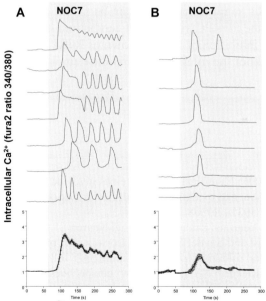

Fig. 1 NO - induced Ca^{2+} signaling in HEK293 cells expressing RyR1. NOC7 (2mM) were applied during each grayed column in the presence (**A**) or the absence (**B**) of extracellular Ca^{2+}. Seven typical recorded traces among individual cells are shown upper and their averaged data (mean ± SEM) on each condition are graphed out below (n=72 cells in **A**, n=32 cells in **B**).

The increments of $[Ca^{2+}]_i$ in the RyR1 – expressing HEK293 cells by NOC7 were in a dose - dependent manner from the Ca^{2+} oscillations to the persistent elevations of $[Ca^{2+}]_i$ observed in individual cells. These Ca^{2+} signals after the application of NOC7 were inhibited by the pretreatment of ryanodine, an open-locked channel blocker of RyRs, but not by ODQ, an sGC inhibitor. These results suggest that the NO can evoke intracellular Ca^{2+} signals through the activation of RyR1 / Ca^{2+} release channels which dose not involve the sGC – PGK pathway. Furthermore, NOC7 could not induce any elevations of $[Ca^{2+}]_i$ in HEK293 cells which expressed the ^{3635}cysteine of RyR1 deficient mutants which did not have the S – nitrosation sites of RyR1 by NO (Aracena – Parks et al. 2006).

3 Conclusion

In this experimental model, we showed that the NO could increase the intracellular Ca^{2+} in living cells through the activation of RyR1 / intracellular Ca^{2+} release channel. The activation of RyR1 by NO required the ^{3635}cysteine of RyR1, which was reported as one of the S-nitrosation site of RyR1. These results suggest that RyR1 can be as one of targets of neurotransmitter NO in the PF - PC synapses of cerebellum in brain. As the next step, PC - specific inhibition or knock - down of RyR1 will be a useful tool for investigation about the roles of RyR1 in the neural plasticity formation of cerebellum.

References

Aracena – Parks P, Goonasekera SA, Gilman CP, Dirksen RT, Hidalgo C and Hamilton SL (2006) Identification of cysteines involved in S – nitrosylation, S – glutathionylation, and oxidation to disulfides in ryanodine receptor type 1. J Biol Chem 281: 40354-40368

Berridge MJ (1998) Neuronal calcium signaling. Neuron 21: 13-26

Bredt DS, Hwang PM and Snyder SH (1990) Localization of nitric oxide synthase indicating a neural role for nitric oxide. Nature 347: 768-770

Edwards TM and Rickard NS (2007) New perspectives on the mechanisms through which nitric oxide may affect learning and memory processes. Neurosci Biobehav Rev. 31: 413-25.

Furuichi T, Furutama D, Hakamata Y, Nakai J, Takeshima H and Mikoshiba K (1994) Multiple types of ryanodine receptor / Ca^{2+} release channels are differentially expressed in rabbit brain. J Neuro Sci 14: 4794-4805

Ignarro LJ and Kadowitz PJ (1985) The pharmacological and physiological role of

cyclic GMP in vascular smooth muscle relaxation. Ann Rev Pharmacol Toxicol 25: 171-191
Lev-Ram V, WongST, Storm DR and Tsien RY (2002) A new form of cerebellar long – term potentiation is postsynaptic and dependent on nitric oxide but not cAMP. Proc Natl Acad Sci USA. 99: 8389-8393
Iino M (2006) Ca^{2+} - dependent inositol 1, 4, 5 – trisphosphate and nitric oxide signaling in cerebellar neurons. J Pharmacol. Sci 100: 538-544
Namiki S, Kakizawa S, Hirose K and Iino M (2005) No signaling decodes frequency of neural activity and generates synapse-specific plasticity in mouse cerebellum. J Physiol 566: 849-863
Zhang J and Snyder SH (1995) Nitric oxide in the nervous system. Ann Rev Pharmacol Toxicol 35:213-233

Decreased sensitivity to negative facial emotions and limbic lesions in patients with myotonic dystrophy type 1

Mitsuru Kawamura,[1,2] Akitoshi Takeda,[1] Mutsutaka Kobayakawa,[1] Atsunobu Suzuki,[3,4,5] Masaki Kondo,[1] and Natsuko Tsuruya,[1]

[1]Department of Neurology, Showa University School of Medicine, 1-5-8 Hatanodai, Shinagawa-ku, Tokyo, 142-8666, Japan

<email> kawa@med.showa-u.ac.jp
[2]Core Research for Evolutional Science and Technology (CREST), Japan Science and Technology Agency (JST), Saitama, Japan
[3]Program of Gerontological Research Organization for Interdisciplinary Research, University of Tokyo, Tokyo, Japan
[4]Beckman Institute, University of Illinois, Urbana, USA
[5]Japan Society for the Promotion of Science

Summary. It has been noted that patients with myotonic dystrophy type 1 (DM 1) exhibit social cognitive impairment. However, the mechanisms of social cognitive functions in DM 1 have not been well examined. We investigated the recognition of facial expressions in patients with DM 1. Four DM 1 patients participated in the experiment. The sensitivity of basic emotions in patients with DM 1 was measured and compared with MRI and SPECT findings. DM 1 patients showed lower sensitivity to fearful, disgusted, and angry faces. DM 1 patients showed lesions in the anterior temporal white matter, the amygdala, the insular, and the orbitofrontal cortex. The sensitivity to facial expressions was decreased in the patients with marked lesions in the anterior temporal area. Patients with relatively mild anterior temporal lesions did not show a significant decrease in sensitivity to facial emotions. The present results indicate subcortical lesions in anterior temporal areas, including the amygdala, the insular, and the orbitofrontal cortex, in some DM 1 patients. Given that the limbic system, including the amygdala, plays an important role in emotional processing, social cognitive impairment in patients with DM 1 could be associated with decreased sensitivity to facial expressions caused by limbic lesions.

Keywords. facial expression, emotion, myotonic dystrophy type 1, social cognition

1 Introduction

Myotonic dystrophy type 1 (DM 1) is a heritable multisystem disease that produces myotonia, amyotrophy, cataract, endocrine disorder, and cardiac myopathy (Machuca-Tzili et al. 2005). Although it has been noted that patients with DM 1 exhibit social cognitive impairment since the time that the disease was identified and named "myotonic dystrophy," the mechanism of social cognitive impairment has not been well examined (Adie and Greenfield 1923; Maas and Paterson 1937). As DM 1 appears in the muscle section of the latest neurology textbook, brain lesions and higher brain function in DM 1 are not focus areas warranting attention.

In recent years, there have been few previous studies examining the mechanism of social cognitive impairment in DM 1 patients. Winblad et al have reported in a well-controlled and multi-case study that DM 1 patients showed impaired facial expression recognition for fear, anger, and disgust (Winblad et al. 2006). However, this study used the forced choice task to examine facial expression recognition, and only two trials were used for each facial expression. Therefore, details of facial expression recognition ability could not be evaluated in the previous study. Furthermore, these results could be confounded by the ceiling effect or the factor of task difficulty for each facial expression.

In the present study, the social cognitive function of DM 1 patients was examined with respect to facial expression recognition. We assessed the sensitivity to facial emotions in DM 1 patients and compared the results with those of magnetic resonance imaging (MRI) and single photon emission computed tomography (SPECT). The results show that sensitivity to facial emotions was decreased in patients with DM 1 and that the decrease was associated with lesions in the limbic system, including the amygdala.

2 Methods

2.1 Participants

Four DM 1 patients were recruited from among outpatients who were diagnosed and regularly treated at the Showa University Hospital. Details of case 1 and 2 were described in elsewhere (Takeda et al. in press). Patients who had a history of mental disease, traumatic brain injury, and alcoholism were not included in the study. DM 1 was diagnosed by the number of CTG repeats (>50) in the DMPK gene on the 19th chromosome.

Additionally, 11 age-, sex-, and education-matched healthy control (HC) subjects participated in the study (7 men and 4 women). They were recruited from a recruiting agency for seniors and were paid for their participation. They had no history of neurological or psychiatric disorders.

Global cognitive function of the participants was assessed using Mini Mental State Examination (MMSE). Depressive state was measured using the Zung Self-Rating Depression Scale (SDS). In the DM 1 patients, visuoperceptual ability and visual memory were assessed using the Rey-Osterrieth Complex Figure test, and executive function was assessed using the Frontal Assessment Battery (FAB).

All patients and control participants were Japanese. A written informed consent was obtained from all participants prior to the beginning of the study. The study was approved by the Showa University Ethics Committee.

2.2 Sensitivity to basic emotions

To investigate facial expression recognition, the method of evaluating "sensitivities to basic emotions in faces" was used (Suzuki et al. 2006). The participants viewed 72 grey-scale photographs of facial expressions and rated the emotional intensity of each facial expression with respect to the six basic emotions: happiness, surprise, fear, anger, disgust, and sadness. The ratings used a 6-point scale from 0 ("not at all") to 5 ("very much"). The stimuli were divided into two sets of 36 photographs: one set consisted of photographs of a Japanese female and the other consisted of photographs of a Caucasian male, "JJ," taken from pictures of facial affect (Ekman and Friesen 1976). In each set of 36 photographs, six were posed, prototypical facial expressions of the six basic emotions and 30 were morphed images of two different prototypical expressions that were created using software for facial image processing (Information-Technology Promotion Agency, Japan, 1998). For each of the 15 possible pairs of the six prototypical expressions, two morphed images were created by blending the prototypical expressions in proportions of 60: 40% and 40: 60%. Each photograph was printed in grey scale on letter-sized glossy photo paper. The order in which the two sets were presented was counterbalanced across the participants. In each set, the order in which the 36 photographs were presented was pseudo-randomized but was identical for all the participants. Each participant's sensitivity to a given emotion was scored by applying the graded-response model (GRM) (Samejima 1970). Because it had been observed that the intensity ratings for surprise did not conform well to the GRM (Suzuki et al, 2005; unpublished work), the study focused on sensitivity to the five basic emotions excluding surprise. See Suzuki et al (2006) for details of the scoring methods(Suzuki et al. 2006).

2.3 Facial expression identification (Kan et al. 2002)

For comparison with the sensitivity task, a conventional test of facial expression recognition was administered, that is, a forced-choice identification (labeling) task of prototypical facial expressions. The test of facial expressions consists of six movies of basic emotions (happiness, sadness, anger, fear, surprise, and disgust) expressed by professional male and female actors. Each emotion was presented twice, first head-on and then from a 45-degree angle. Consequently, there were 6 (emotions) × 2 (male and female) × 2 (head-on and 45-degree angle) = 24 stimuli. The videotapes had no sound, to ensure that the facial expressions were the only indicator of emotional state.

2.4 Facial identity matching

The participants were asked to match a facial photograph (target) to an array of six facial photographs (references) of different persons of the same gender. The photographs used in this task were selected from the Facial Information Norm Database (Yoshida et al. 2004) (FIND) distributed by Nihon University. The matching involved three conditions (i.e., Test 1, a front-view target with front-view references; Test 2, a front-view target with side-view references; and Test 3, an upward target with front-view references); each condition included 10 trials. The 30 trials, consisting of a target and six references, were presented to the participants in either of two pseudo-randomized orders and the orders assigned were counterbalanced across participants.

2.5 Assessment of brain lesions

To examine structural abnormalities in the brain, MR images were obtained using a 1.5 T MR imager (Genesis Signa; General Electric, Milwaukee, WI, USA or Magnetom Vision; Siemens, Germany). T2-weighted axial slices were obtained throughout the whole brain (TR: repetition time/TE: echo time = 3800-4920/96 ms, thickness 5 mm) and fluid-attenuated inversion recovery (FLAIR) imaging coronal slices were obtained throughout the whole brain (TR/TE/inversion time: TI = 7000-8002/108-110/2000 ms, thickness 6 mm). To examine cerebral perfusion, ^{99m}Tc-ethyl Cysteinate Dimer single photon emission computed tomography (ECD-SPECT) images were also obtained using a double-headed rotating gamma camera (ECAM, Siemens) equipped with a parallel hole collimator. Patients were injected with 600 MBq of ECD intravenously in a resting state with their eyes closed. The SPECT scanning started 5 minutes after injection. These images were obtained for all DM 1 patients at the time of facial expression evaluation. The lesions were interpreted by experienced neurologists (A.T., Ma.K., and Mi.K.).

3 Results

3.1 Neuropsychological tests

DM 1 patients did not exhibit severe impairment in intellectual, visuospatial, or frontal lobe functions compared with normal participants. The SDS scores of the patients were also in the normal range, although higher than those of HC subjects (Table 1).

3.2 Sensitivity to basic emotions

Regarding sensitivity to facial emotions, the pattern of results was different between Cases 1 and 2 and Cases 3 and 4 (Figure 1). Cases 1 and 2 displayed lower sensitivity scores than the HC subjects for all emotions except happiness. Sensitivity scores were significantly lower for anger and disgust in Case 1 ($P = 0.04$, z = -2.11 and $P = 0.03$, z = -2.22, respectively) and for disgust and fear in Case 2 ($P = 0.008$, z = -2.67 and $P = 0.005$, z = -2.78, respectively). Meanwhile, sensitivity scores were in the normal range for Cases 3 and 4.

Table 1. Participant characteristics

		Case 1	Case 2	Case 3	Case 4	HC mean (SD)
Age		35	55	62	74	51.4 (10.9)
Sex		M	F	M	F	M:F = 7:4
Years of education		12	9	16	12	16.8 (8.73)
Disease duration		25	19	12	1	–
Age at onset		10	36	50	73	–
CTG Repeats		1300	1300	70	70	–
MMSE		24	29	24	24	29.6 (0.7)
FAB		13	14	12	12	–
ROCFT	Copy	19	22	34	–	–
	Recall	18.5	5	14	–	–
SDS		33	52	57	49	38.5 (8.73)
FIM	Test 1	10	10	10	10	9.7 (0.6)
	Test 2	9	9	8	10	9.1 (1.4)
	Test 3	4	3	6	4	6.7 (1.6)

HC, Healthy Controls; SD, Standard Deviation; MMSE, Mini Mental State Examination; FAB, Frontal Assessment Battery; ROCFT, Rey-Osterrieth Complex Figure test; SDS, Zung Self-Rating Depression Scale; FIM, Facial Identity Matching test

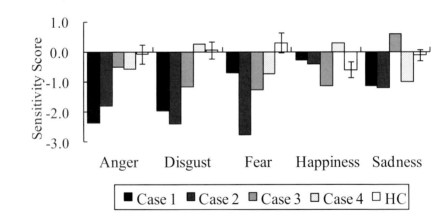

Figure 1. Sensitivity Scores (Means) for the DM 1 Patients and Healthy Controls (HC). Error bars represent standard errors. Compared with HC subjects, sensitivity scores were lower for angry and disgusted faces for Case 1, and for disgusted and fearful faces for Case 2. Sensitivity scores were in the normal range for Cases 3 and 4.

3.3 Facial expression identification

The number of correct responses is shown in Table 2. DM 1 patients could discriminate facial emotions as well as HC subjects.

3.4 Facial identity matching

Although scores for facial identity matching were lower in the DM 1 patients compared to HC patients, the difference was not statistically significant except for Case 2 in discriminating upward and front-view faces (Table 1, Test 3). DM 1 patients tended to make errors in discriminating faces seen from an unfamiliar view (Test 3), while face recognition in normal views (Tests 1 and 2) was relatively unaffected.

3.5 MRI and SPECT

All the DM 1 patients exhibited high-intensity areas in cerebral white matter on T2 weighted and FLAIR images. However, the distribution and intensity of the lesions were different between Cases 1 and 2 and Cases 3 and 4. In Cases 1 and 2, high signal areas were mainly located in bilateral anterior temporal areas, including subcortical white matter, the amygdala, and entorhinal cortex (Figure 2). Lesions were also found in the insular and the orbitofrontal cortex. Although Cases 3 and 4 showed high intensity areas in the insular and the orbitofrontal cortex, intensity in the anterior temporal areas was not so prominent.

Similar results were obtained in the SPECT imaging. Cases 1 and 2 showed hypoperfusion in bilateral anterior and medial temporal cortexes and the orbitofrontal cortex. These areas were consistent with the lesions found in MRI. However, Cases 3 and 4 did not exhibit marked hypoperfusion.

Table 2. Results for facial expression identification

	Case 1	Case 2	Case 3	Case 4	HC mean (SD)
Anger	1.0	1.0	1.0	1.0	0.98 (0.05)
Disgust	1.0	1.0	1.0	1.0	0.94 (0.12)
Fear	0.75	0.75	1.0	1.0	0.83 (0.2)
Sadness	1.0	1.0	0.75	1.0	1.0 (0.0)
Happiness	1.0	1.0	1.0	1.0	1.0 (0.0)
Surprise	1.0	1.0	1.0	1.0	0.96 (0.08)

SD, Standard Deviation

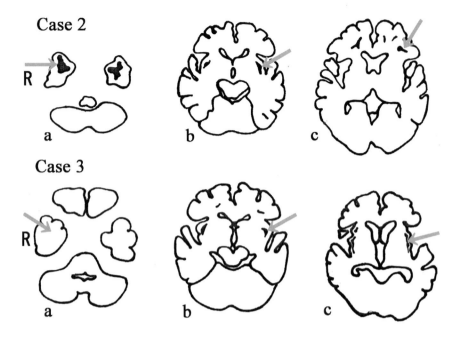

Figure 2. The Distribution of Brain Lesions in Cases 2 and 3.
In the MRI results, Case 2 showed high signal areas mainly in bilateral anterior temporal areas, including subcortical white matter, the amygdala, and the entorhinal cortex. Lesions were also found in the insular and the orbitofrontal cortex. MRI of Case 1 showed similar patterns to that of Case 2. Case 3 showed high intensity areas in the insular and the orbitofrontal cortex, while signal intensities in the anterior temporal subcortex were not so prominent in MRI. MRI of Case 4 showed similar patterns to that of Case 3.

4 Discussion

4.1 Decreased sensitivity to facial emotions

Decreased sensitivity to facial emotions in DM 1 patients was revealed using a refined assessment method in which difficulty factors were controlled (Suzuki et al. 2006). In patients with DM 1, the sensitivity score was significantly lower for anger, sadness, fear, and disgust. Lower sensitivity to facial emotions was found in the patients with subcortical lesions in temporal areas, including the amygdala. Although Case 2 showed difficulty in discriminating upward and front-view faces, visual impairment could not explain the lower sensitivity to facial emotions, since the patients could discriminate front-view faces in the facial identity matching test.

As shown in the facial expression identification task in the present study, it is not easy to detect the impairment of facial expression recognition in DM 1 patients using a conventional task. A refined assessment method was developed in which difficulty factors were controlled by means of mixed facial expressions (Suzuki et al. 2006). The refined task allows detection of sensitivity to each basic emotion without being confounded by task difficulties. Moreover, use of this task permits detection of decreased sensitivity to facial emotions in a single case. Patients with lesions in the anterior temporal subcortex (Cases 1 and 2) showed decreased sensitivity to negative emotions, while patients without the lesions (Cases 3 and 4) did not. These results indicate that impaired facial expression recognition was associated with subcortex white matter lesions, especially in the anterior temporal subcortex.

4.2 Brain lesions

Cases 1 and 2 exhibited subcortical lesions in the bilateral anterior temporal areas, including the amygdala and the entorhinal cortex. These lesions were observed in patients with a greater number of CTG repeats. Cases 3 and 4 did not exhibit the marked lesions in the anterior temporal cortex that Cases 1 and 2 did, although they exhibited lesions in the insular cortex and the orbitofrontal cortex.

The anatomical findings in the present study are consistent with previous studies. DM 1 has been reported to be associated with white matter lesions and cortical atrophy in the temporal pole and periventricle in MRI (Bachmann et al. 1996; Kornblum et al. 2004) and hypoperfusion in the frontal, temporal, cingulate, and orbitofrontal cortex in SPECT (Chang et al. 1993; Meola et al. 2003). Autopsy studies of DM 1 patients showed decreased myelin sheaths and severely disordered arrangement of axons in anterior temporal white matter, which disrupted the white matter connections between the anterior temporal cortex and the amygdala (Ogata et al. 1998). Neurofibrillary tangles were found in the entorhinal cortex, the hippocampus, the amygdala, and in most of the temporal areas (Yoshimura et al. 1990; Vermersch et al. 1996; Oyamada et al. 2006). The MRI and SPECT findings in the present study probably reflected these pathological changes in DM 1 patients.

4.3 Facial expression recognition and amygdala lesions

Neural mechanisms of social cognitive impairment and personality in DM 1 have not been well addressed. The present study shows that impairment in facial expression recognition was associated with lesions in the anterior temporal subcortex, which coincided with the circuit for emotional processing (Yakovlev 1948; Nauta 1962). Previous MRI/SPECT studies on DM 1 patients have mainly focused attention on the relationship between these lesions and intellectual or frontal lobe functions (Chang et al. 1993; Meola et al. 2003). While there are a few studies that associated temporal lesions with CTG repeats, intelligence, or disease duration, no study has indicated the association between anterior temporal lesions and facial expression recognition (Huber et al. 1989; Di Costanzo et al. 2001; Kuo et al. 2008). Winblad et al found a correlation between the ability to recognize facial expressions and CTG repeats (Winblad et al. 2006). However, they did not fully address the relationship between brain lesions and facial expression recognition in DM 1 patients. The present results suggest that anterior temporal lesions in DM 1 patients result in dysfunction of emotional processing, appearing as impairment of facial expression recognition. We consider that the anterior temporal lesions result in the amygdala dysfunctions in DM 1. Insensitivity to the negative facial emotions in cases with anterior temporal lesions is consistent with the previous reports that showed the amygdala is associated with recognition of facial emotions, especially for negative facial expressions (Adolphs et al. 1994; Adolphs et al. 1995; Adolphs et al. 1999; Yoshimura et al. 2005). An increase in CTG repeats may, by producing anterior temporal subcortex lesions, be related to impaired facial expression recognition.

The present study indicating decreased sensitivity to facial emotions in patients with DM 1 is considered to reflect a dysfunction of the limbic system, including the amygdala. Decreased sensitivity to negative emotions may possibly account for social cognitive impairment. Social cognitive impairment in DM 1 has been discussed in terms of personality dysfunction (Adie and Greenfield 1923; Maas and Paterson 1937). Patients with DM 1 have been reported to be less cooperative and empathetic (Winblad et al. 2005). Social cognitive impairment in DM 1 patients could be attributed to decreased sensitivity to negative facial emotions, caused by limbic lesions.

Acknowledgements

M.K. was supported by a grant from Core Research for Evolutional Science and Technology (CREST, 17022035) and the Grant-in-Aid for Scientific Research on Priority Areas—System study on higher-order brain functions from the Ministry of Education, Culture, Sports, Science and Technology (MEXT, 18020027). This study was also supported in part by a Showa University Grant-in-Aid for Innovative Collaborative Research Projects and a Special Research Grant-in-Aid for Development of Characteristic Education from MEXT.

References

Adie W, Greenfield J (1923). "Dystrophia myotonica (myotonia atrophica)." Brain 46: 73-127.
Adolphs R, Tranel D, Damasio H, Damasio A (1994). "Impaired recognition of emotion in facial expressions following bilateral damage to the human amygdala." Nature 372(6507): 669-672.
Adolphs R, Tranel D, Damasio H, Damasio AR (1995). "Fear and the human amygdala." J. Neurosci. 15(9): 5879-5891.
Adolphs R, Tranel D, Hamann S, Young AW, Calder AJ, Phelps EA, Anderson A, Lee GP, Damasio AR (1999). "Recognition of facial emotion in nine individuals with bilateral amygdala damage." Neuropsychologia 37(10): 1111-1117.
Bachmann G, Damian MS, Koch M, Schilling G, Fach B, Stoppler S (1996). "The clinical and genetic correlates of MRI findings in myotonic dystrophy." Neuroradiology 38(7): 629-635.
Chang L, Anderson T, Migneco OA, Boone K, Mehringer CM, Villanueva-Meyer J, Berman N, Mena I (1993). "Cerebral abnormalities in myotonic dystrophy. Cerebral blood flow, magnetic resonance imaging, and neuropsychological tests." Arch. Neurol. 50(9): 917-923.
Di Costanzo A, Di Salle F, Santoro L, Bonavita V, Tedeschi G (2001). "T2 relaxometry of brain in myotonic dystrophy." Neuroradiology 43(3): 198-204.
Ekman P, Friesen W (1976). Pictures of facial affect. Palo Alto, CA, Consulting Psychologists Press.
Huber SJ, Kissel JT, Shuttleworth EC, Chakeres DW, Clapp LE, Brogan MA (1989). "Magnetic resonance imaging and clinical correlates of intellectual impairment in myotonic dystrophy." Arch. Neurol. 46(5): 536-540.
Kan Y, Kawamura M, Hasegawa Y, Mochizuki S, Nakamura K (2002). "Recognition of emotion from facial, prosodic and written verbal stimuli in Parkinson's disease." Cortex 38(4): 623-630.
Kornblum C, Reul J, Kress W, Grothe C, Amanatidis N, Klockgether T, Schroder R (2004). "Cranial magnetic resonance imaging in genetically proven myotonic dystrophy type 1 and 2." J. Neurol. 251(6): 710-714.
Kuo HC, Hsieh YC, Wang HM, Chuang WL, Huang CC (2008). "Correlation among subcortical white matter lesions, intelligence and CTG repeat expansion in classic myotonic dystrophy type 1." Acta Neurol. Scand. 117(2): 101-107.

Maas O, Paterson A (1937). "Mental changes in families affected by dystrophia myotonica." Lancet 1: 21-23.

Machuca-Tzili L, Brook D, Hilton-Jones D (2005). "Clinical and molecular aspects of the myotonic dystrophies: a review." Muscle Nerve 32(1): 1-18.

Meola G, Sansone V, Perani D, Scarone S, Cappa S, Dragoni C, Cattaneo E, Cotelli M, Gobbo C, Fazio F, Siciliano G, Mancuso M, Vitelli E, Zhang S, Krahe R, Moxley RT (2003). "Executive dysfunction and avoidant personality trait in myotonic dystrophy type 1 (DM-1) and in proximal myotonic myopathy (PROMM/DM-2)." Neuromuscul. Disord. 13(10): 813-821.

Nauta W (1962). "Neural associations of the amygdaloid complex in the monkey." Brain 85: 505-520.

Ogata A, Terae S, Fujita M, Tashiro K (1998). "Anterior temporal white matter lesions in myotonic dystrophy with intellectual impairment: an MRI and neuropathological study." Neuroradiology 40(7): 411-415.

Oyamada R, Hayashi M, Katoh Y, Tsuchiya K, Mizutani T, Tominaga I, Kashima H (2006). "Neurofibrillary tangles and deposition of oxidative products in the brain in cases of myotonic dystrophy." Neuropathology 26(2): 107-114.

Samejima F (1970). "Estimation of latent ability using a response pattern of graded scores." Psychometrika 35(1): 139.

Suzuki A, Hoshino T, Shigemasu K (2006). "Measuring individual differences in sensitivities to basic emotions in faces." Cognition 99: 327-353.

Suzuki A, Hoshino T, Shigemasu K, Kawamura M (2006). "Disgust-specific impairment of facial expression recognition in Parkinson's disease." Brain 129(Pt 3): 707-717.

Takeda A, Kobayakawa M, Suzuki A, Tsuruya N, Kawamura M (in press). "Lowered sensitivity to facial emotions in Myotonic Dystrophy Type 1." J. Neurol. Sci.

Vermersch P, Sergeant N, Ruchoux MM, Hofmann-Radvanyi H, Wattez A, Petit H, Dwailly P, Delacourte A (1996). "Specific tau variants in the brains of patients with myotonic dystrophy." Neurology 47(3): 711-717.

Winblad S, Hellstrom P, Lindberg C, Hansen S (2006). "Facial emotion recognition in myotonic dystrophy type 1 correlates with CTG repeat expansion." J. Neurol. Neurosurg. Psychiatry 77(2): 219-223.

Winblad S, Lindberg C, Hansen S (2005). "Temperament and character in patients with classical myotonic dystrophy type 1 (DM-1)." Neuromuscul. Disord. 15(4): 287-292.

Yakovlev P (1948). "Motility, Behavior, and the Brain: Stereodynamic organization and neural coordinates of behavior." J. Nerv. Ment. Dis. 107: 313-335.

Yoshida H, Suzuki R, Watanabe N, Yamaguchi T, Ogawa Y, Kitamura M, Maeda A, Tsuzuki D, Tokita G, Wada M, Morishima S, Yamada H (2004). "The second report of constructing facial information norm database: capturing environment and searching interface of images." IEIC Technical Report 104(198(HCS2004 10-17)): 13-16.

Yoshimura N, Kawamura M, Masaoka Y, Homma I (2005). "The amygdala of patients with Parkinson's disease is silent in response to fearful facial expressions." Neuroscience 131(2): 523-534.

Yoshimura N, Otake M, Igarashi K, Matsunaga M, Takebe K, Kudo H (1990). "Topography of Alzheimer's neurofibrillary change distribution in myotonic dystrophy." Clin. Neuropathol. 9(5): 234-239.

Generation of Rac1 conditional mutant mice by Cre/loxP system

Dai Suzuki[1], Atsushi Yamada[1], Takanori Amano[2], Ayako Kimura[3], Rika Yasuhara[1], Mizuho Sakahara[4], Masaru Tamura[2], Noriyuki Tsumaki[5], Shu Takeda[3], Masanori Nakamura[6], Toshihiko Shiroishi[2], Atsu Aiba[4], Ryutaro Kamijo[1]

Departments of [1]Biochemistry and [6]Oral Anatomy and Developmental Biology, School of Dentistry, Showa University, 1-5-8 Hatanodai, Shinagawa, Tokyo 142-8555, Japan, [2]Mouse Genomics Resource Laboratory, National Institute of Genetics, 1111 Yata, Mishima, Shizuoka 411-0801, Japan, [3]Department of Orthopedic Surgery, Graduate School, Tokyo Medical and Dental University 1-5-45 Yushima, Bunkyo, Tokyo 113-8519, Japan, [4]Division of Molecular Biology, Department of Biochemistry and Molecular Biology, Kobe University Graduate School of Medicine, 7-5-1 Kusunoki-cho, Chuo-ku, Kobe 650-0017, Japan, [5]Department of Bone and Cartilage Biology, Osaka University Graduate School of Medicine, 2-2 Yamadaoka, Suita, Osaka 565-0871, Japan

Summary. Rac1 is a small GTPase which belongs to the Rho family of proteins, and has multiple roles in cellular function, including actin cytoskeleton organization, transcriptional activation, microtubule formation, and endocytosis. In the present study, the mesenchyme of mouse limbs was made deficient in Rac1 in order to investigate its role in digit morphogenesis during limb development. We employed a Cre-loxP system for limb bud mesenchyme-specific inactivation of the *Rac1* gene, as null mice show embryonic lethality.

Key words. Rac1, Cre-loxP system, limb bud mesenchyme

1 Introduction

The Rho family of small GTPases regulates the cytoskeleton and transcription by virtue of cycling between inactive GDP-bound and active GTP-bound forms (Hall, 1994). The Rac subfamily consists of Rac1, Rac2, and Rac3, and they participate in a wide range of cellular functions, such as actin cytoskeletal reorganization (Ridley et al., 1992), cell adhesion (Hall, 1998), cell growth (Olson et al., 1995), and superoxide formation (Mizuno et al., 1992). However, the tissue-specific roles of Rac1 in mammalian growth and development in vivo remain largely unknown.

Herein, we describe the generation of limb mesenchymal cell-specific inactivation of the *Rac1* gene in mice.

2 Materials and Methods

2.1 Generation of Rac1 conditional mutant mice

Rac1 alleles were used in this study. The first exon was flanked by loxP sites (flox) and deleted upon Cre-mediated recombination, causing the deletion of the exon1 allele, which is functionally equivalent to a null (Kassai et al., 2008). Rac1 conditional mutant mice were generated by mating *Rac1* flox mice ($Rac1^{flox/flox}$) with *Prx1-Cre* transgenic (*Prx1-Cre* Tg) mice (Logan et al., 2002).

2.2 Genotyping

Genotypes were assessed by PCR analysis using appropriate primer pairs (Table 1).

3 Results and Discussion

For the present study, we employed a Cre-loxP system for limb bud mesenchyme-specific inactivation of the *Rac1* gene, as *Rac1* null mice develop embryonic lethal. Mice with a conditional (floxed) mutation in both alleles of the *Rac1* gene ($Rac1^{flox/flox}$) were crossed with mice expressing

Table 1. The primer sequences used for PCR analysis

Primers	Direction	Sequence (5'-3')
Rac1	Sense primer	ATTTTCTAGATTCCACTTGTGAAC
	Antisense primer	ATCCCTACTTCCTTCCAACTC
Cre	Sense primer	GACGATGCAACGAGTGATGA
	Antisense primer	AGCATTGCTGTCACTTGGTC

The reaction conditions for all PCRs were 30 cycles of denaturation at 94℃ for 30 s, annealing at 58℃ for 30 s, and extension at 72℃ for 30 s.

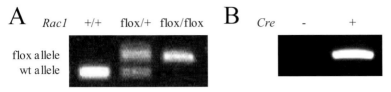

Fig. 1. Representative PCR genotyping reactions.
(A) The wild-type (wt) and floxed (flox) alleles of *Rac1* were detected by PCR using the primers indicated in Table 1. Genomic DNA was isolated from the tails of mice with genotypes $Rac1^{+/+}$, $Rac1^{flox/+}$, and $Rac1^{flox/flox}$. (B) PCR for the *Prx1-Cre* transgene (*Cre*) was performed using tail extracts of *Prx1-Cre* (-) and *Prx1-Cre* (+) mice.

Cre recombinase under the control of a *Prx1* limb enhancer (*Prx1-Cre* Tg) to obtain $Rac1^{flox/+}$/*Prx1-Cre* Tg mice. Then, $Rac1^{flox/+}$/*Prx1-Cre* Tg males were crossed with $Rac1^{flox/flox}$ females to obtain $Rac1^{flox/flox}$/*Prx1-Cre* Tg mice, to prevent the carryover of Cre recombinase in the cytoplasm of the oocyte (Ovchinnikov *et al.*, 2006). Genotypes of *Rac1* alleles ($Rac1^{+/+}$, $Rac1^{flox/+}$, $Rac1^{flox/flox}$) and the *Prx1-Cre* transgene were determined by PCR analysis (Fig. 1A, B).

Wang G. *et al.* demonstrated that the cartilage specific inactivation of Rac1 in vivo using mouse Collagen II promoter-driven Cre-expressing transgenic (*Col2-Cre* Tg) mice resulted in increased lethality, skeletal deformities, severe kyphosis, and dwarfism, which suggest that Rac1 is required for endochondral bone development (Wang *et al.*, 2007). However, the expression of Cre in *Col2-Cre* Tg is observed later in the limbs, after mesenchymal cells have committed to a chondrocyte lineage, while the perichondrium is not efficiently targeted (Terpstra *et al.*, 2003). Logan *et al*, showed that *Prx1-Cre* is active in the emerging forelimb bud mesenchyme at E9.5 and hindlimb mesenchyme at E10.5 (Logan *et al.*, 2002). Comparisons of the phenotype of these two mouse models suggest the spacious and temporal roles of Rac1 in embryonic endochondral bone formation during limb development.

In summary, the ablation of Rac1 in limb bud mesenchymal cells may provide new insights into limb development.

4 Acknowledgments

We are grateful to Dr. N Wada for critical discussion and Dr. T Sagai for technical support. This work was supported in part by the 'High-Tech Research Center' Project for Private Universities, a matching fund subsidy from the Ministry of Education, Culture, Sports, Science and Technology of Japan, and Grants-in-Aid for Scientific research from the Japan Society for the Promotion of Science.

5 References

Hall, A. (1994). Small GTP-binding proteins and the regulation of the actin cytoskeleton. Annu Rev Cell Biol 10, 31-54.

Hall, A. (1998). Rho GTPases and the actin cytoskeleton. Science 279, 509-14.

Kassai, H., Terashima, T., Fukaya, M., Nakao, K., Sakahara, M., Watanabe, M. and Aiba, A. (2008). Rac1 in cortical projection neurons is selectively required for midline crossing of commissural axonal formation. Eur J Neurosci 28, 257-67.

Logan, M., Martin, J. F., Nagy, A., Lobe, C., Olson, E. N. and Tabin, C. J. (2002). Expression of Cre Recombinase in the developing mouse limb bud driven by a Prxl enhancer. Genesis 33, 77-80.

Mizuno, T., Kaibuchi, K., Ando, S., Musha, T., Hiraoka, K., Takaishi, K., Asada, M., Nunoi, H., Matsuda, I. and Takai, Y. (1992). Regulation of the superoxide-generating NADPH oxidase by a small GTP-binding protein and its stimulatory and inhibitory GDP/GTP exchange proteins. J Biol Chem 267, 10215-8.

Olson, M. F., Ashworth, A. and Hall, A. (1995). An essential role for Rho, Rac, and Cdc42 GTPases in cell cycle progression through G1. Science 269, 1270-2.

Ovchinnikov, D. A., Selever, J., Wang, Y., Chen, Y. T., Mishina, Y., Martin, J. F. and Behringer, R. R. (2006). BMP receptor type IA in limb bud mesenchyme regulates distal outgrowth and patterning. Dev Biol 295, 103-15.

Ridley, A. J., Paterson, H. F., Johnston, C. L., Diekmann, D. and Hall, A. (1992). The small GTP-binding protein rac regulates growth factor-induced membrane ruffling. Cell 70, 401-10.

Terpstra, L., Prud'homme, J., Arabian, A., Takeda, S., Karsenty, G., Dedhar, S. and St-Arnaud, R. (2003). Reduced chondrocyte proliferation and chondrodysplasia in mice lacking the integrin-linked kinase in chondrocytes. J Cell Biol 162, 139-48.

Wang, G., Woods, A., Agoston, H., Ulici, V., Glogauer, M. and Beier, F. (2007). Genetic ablation of Rac1 in cartilage results in chondrodysplasia. Dev Biol 306, 612-23.

Orexin modulates neuronal activities of mesencephalic trigeminal sensory neurons in rats

Kiyomi Nakayama, Ayako Mochizuki, Shiro Nakamura, Tomio Inoue

Department of Oral Physiology, Showa University School of Dentistry, 1-5-8 Hatanodai, Shinagawa-ku, Tokyo 142-8555, Japan
<e-mail> inouet@dent.showa-u.ac.jp

Summary. Orexin is a regulatory peptide involved in the control of feeding, motivation and adaptive behaviors. To examine the role of orexin in mastication, whole cell patch-clamp recordings from mesencephalic trigeminal sensory neurons (Mes V neurons), which are critical components of the circuits controlling oral-motor activity, were performed on brainstem slice preparations from Wistar rats aged between postnatal days (P) 0-17. By bath-application of orexin-A (200-500 nM), small membrane depolarizations with decreases of the input resistance were observed at the resting potential in the presence of tetrodotoxin. In rats older than P7 or P8, it is known that the burst discharges are induced by a depolarizing step pulse at a holding potential of about -40 to -50 mV in Mes V neurons. Such conditional burst discharges in Mes V neurons were reduced to 61% of control by bath-application of orexin-A. Persistent sodium currents, which contribute to production of such conditional burst discharges, were also reduced by orexin-A. These results suggest that orexin modulates oral-motor behavior via Mes V neurons.

Key words. Orexin, Mesencephalic trigeminal sensory neuron, Whole cell patch-clamp recording, rat

1 Introduction

Orexin-A and orexin-B are a pair of neuro peptides derived from a common precursor peptide, the product of the prepro-orexin (de Lecea et al. 1998, Sakurai et al. 1998). The actions of orexins are mediated by two G protein-coupled receptors termed orexin receptor type 1 and orexin receptor type 2. Orexin-containing neurons project from the lateral hypothalamic area, a region of the brain implicated in feeding, arousal, and motivated behavior, to numerous brain regions, with the limbic system, hypothalamus, and monoaminergic and cholinergic nuclei of brainstem receiving particularly strong innervations. Thus, the orexinergic system is anatomically well placed to influence the feeding, arousal, motivational, metabolic, autonomic behaviors.

Recently, the orexin receptor type 1 has been detected in Mes V neurons using immunohistochemical techniques (S. Sioda, unpublished observation). Mes V neurons are primary sensory neurons with cell bodies within the nervous system. They relay sensory inputs from the jaw-closer muscle spindles and periodontal mechanoreceptors to trigeminal jaw-closer motoneurons, interneurons, and other brainstem nuclei (Appenteng et al. 1985).

In this study, we tested the effects of orexin-A, which is an agonist of the orexin receptor type 1, on physiological properties in Mes V neurons.

2 Material and methods

Transverse brainstem slices (300-500 μm) were obtained from neonatal and juvenile Wistar rats (P0-17). Mes V neurons were identified by the localization and the morphological features under infrared video microscopy with differential interference contrast, and whole cell patch-clamp recordings were made from Mes V neurons. Current-clamp experiments were performed with an internal solution of (in mM) 140 K-gluconate, 10 KCl, 2 $MgCl_2$, 2 ATP-Na_2, 0.3 GTP-Na_2, 2 spermine, 10 HEPES, 0.2 EGTA. For the recording of sodium currents in voltage-clamp experiments, electrodes were filled with a solution of (in mM) 130 CsF, 9 NaCl, 10 HEPES, 10 EGTA 1 $MgCl_2$, 3 K_2-ATP, 1 Na-GTP. ACSF contained (in mM) 130 NaCl, 3 KCl, 2 $CaCl_2$, 2 $MgCl_2$, 1.25 NaH_2PO_4, 26 $NaHCO_3$, 10 glucose.

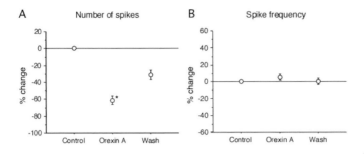

Fig. 1. Effects of orexin-A application on number of spikes **(A)** and spike frequency **(B)** of the conditional burst discharges. *$P < 0.01$ vs control

3 Results

To examine whether orexin-A affects the resting membrane potential in Mes V neurons, current clamp recordings were made from Mes V neurons. By bath-application of Orexin A (500 nM), small membrane depolarizations to < 3 mV with decreases of the input resistance were observed at the resting membrane potential. The orexin-induced membrane depolarization was not affected by the presence of tetrodotoxin (1 μM). The membrane depolarization was increased with postnatal development. The mean membrane depolarizations were 0.23 ± 0.51 mV at P0-3 (n = 5), 1.20 ± 0.28 mV at P8-11 (n = 13), 2.87 ± 1.09 mV at P16-17 (n = 4). The membrane depolarization at P16-17 was significantly larger than at P0-3 ($P < 0.01$).

In rats older than P7 or P8, it is known that conditional burst discharges are induced by a depolarizing step pulse at a holding potential of about -40 to -50 mV in Mes V neurons (Wu et al. 2001). To examine whether orexin-A affects the conditional burst discharges, current-clamp recordings were made from Mes V neurons at a depolarized holding potential of -45 mV. The 0.5-0.8 nA depolarization pulse induced the long lasting burst discharges for 200-930 msec. Bath-application of orexin-A (200 nM) reduced the conditional burst discharges in Mes V neurons. The spike numbers of the conditional burst discharges were significantly reduced to $61 \pm 5\%$ of control by orexin-A (n = 11, $P < 0.01$, Fig. 1A), although the spike frequencies were not affected by orexin-A (Fig. 1B).

It is known that persistent sodium currents contribute to production of the conditional burst discharges (Wu et al. 2005). We examined whether the persistent sodium currents in Mes V neurons change by application of orexin-A. The persistent sodium currents were evoked by a slow voltage ramp protocol (33.3 mV/s) in the presence of TEA (20 mM), 4-AP (1 mM) and Cd^{2+} (0.3 mM) using the voltage-clamp methods. The peak persistent sodium currents were significantly reduced by 30 ± 4% by bath-application of orexin-A (200 nM) (n = 5, $P < 0.01$). These results suggest that the decrease of the persistent sodium currents is responsible for the decrease of the conditional burst discharges by orexin-A in Mes V neurons.

4 Discussion

In this study, we show that orexin-A affects the burst discharge pattern in Mes V neurons via regulations of the persistent sodium currents. Mes V neurons are primary sensory neurons, which play important roles in production of appropriate jaw movements (Morimoto et al. 1989). It is likely that orexin modulates oral-motor behavior via mesencephalic trigeminal neurons.

References

Appenteng K, Donga R, Williams RG (1985) Morphological and electrophysiological determination of the projections of jaw-elevator muscle spindle afferents in rats. J Physiol 369:93-113

de Lecea L, Kilduff TS, Peyron C, Gao X, Foye PE, Danielson PE, Fukuhara C, Battenberg EL, Gautvik VT, Bartlett II FS, Frankel WN, van den Pol AN, Bloom FE, Gautvik KM, Sutcliffe JG (1998) The hypocretins: hypothalamus-specific peptides with neuroexcitatory activity. Proc Natl Acad Sci USA 95:322-327

Morimoto T, Inoue T, Masuda Y, Nagashima T (1989) Sensory components facilitating jaw-closing muscle activities in the rabbit. Exp Brain Res 76:424-440

Sakurai T, Amemiya A, Ishii M, Matsuzaki I, Chemelli RM, Tanaka H, Williams SC, Richardson JA, Kozlowski GP, Wilson S, Arch JR, Buckingham RE, Haynes AC, Carr SA, Annan RS, McNulty DE, Liu WS, Terrett JA, Elshourbagy NA, Bergsma DJ, Yanagisawa M (1998) Orexins and orexin receptors: a family of hypothalamic neuropeptides and G protein-coupled receptors that regulate feeding behavior. Cell 92:573-585

Wu N, Hsiao CF, Chandler SH (2001) Membrane resonance and subthreshold membrane oscillations in mesencephalic V neurons: participants in burst generation. J Neurosci 21:3729-3739

Wu N, Enomoto A, Tanaka S, Hsiao CF, Nykamp DQ, Izhikevich E, Chandler SH (2005) Persistent sodium currents in mesencephalic v neurons participate in burst generation and control of membrane excitability. J Neurophysiol 93:2710-2722.

Investigation of the anxiolytic effects of Kampo formulation, Kamishoyosan, used for treating menopausal psychotic syndromes in women

Kazuo Toriizuka[1], Yumiko Hori[1], Motonori Fukumura[1], Susumu Isoda[2], Yasuaki Hirai[2] and Yoshiteru Ida[1,3]

[1] Laboratory of Pharmacognosy and Phytochemistry, School of Pharmacy
Showa University, Hatanodai, Shinagawa-ku, Tokyo 142-8555, Japan
[2] Laboratory of Herbal Garden, School of Pharmacy
Showa University, Hatanodai, Shinagawa-ku, Tokyo 142-8555, Japan
[3] Yokohama College of Pharmacy, 601 Matano-cho, Totsuka-ku, Yokohama 245-0066, Japan
<e-mail> k-tori@pharm.showa-u.ac.jp

Summary. The anxiolytic effects of four Kampo formulations (Japanese traditional herbal medicines): Tokishakuyakusan, Kamishoyosan, Keishibukuryogan, and Unkeito, were investigated. These Kampo formulations ware used to treat menopausal syndromes in women. Although the herbal ingredients of each Kampo formula are similar, clinical uses of these Kampo formulations are different. Therefore we investigate the differences of them from the basic pharmacological and chemical studies.

From the comparative study of these Kampo formulations, we found the anxiolytic effects of Kamishoyosan (KSS), consists of ten crude herbal drugs. KSS and its composed herbs were assessed by the social interaction (SI) test in mice. Oral administration of KSS dose-dependently increased the SI time. The effect of KSS on SI time was significantly blocked by the gamma-amino-butyric acid A / benzodiazepine (GABA$_A$/BZP) receptor antagonist flumazenil. In addition, 5α-reductase inhibitor finasteride markedly blocked the effect of KSS. When the extract of KSS minus Gardeniae Fructus (the formulae excluding Gardeniae Fructus) was administered, the anxiolytic effect was significantly decreased. On the other hand, the administration of the extract of Gardeniae Fructus or genipiside, major chemical component, increased the SI time. The anxiolytic effect of geniposide was also blocked by flumazenil and finasteride. These findings suggest that Gardeniae Fructus and geniposide have important roles in the anxiolytic effect of KSS, and their anxiolytic effects are mediated by $GABA_A$/BZP receptor stimulation involved in the neurosteroids synthesis.

Key Words. anxiolytic, Gardeniae Fructus, Kampo medicines, neurosteroid, social interaction test

1 Introduction

Around the age of menopause, most women are likely to experience general malaise (known as 'menopausal syndromes'), including mental disorders such as anxiety, insomnia, irritability and depression. Although the mechanisms underlying menopausal mental disorders are unclear, the decline of ovarian steroids seems to produce some functional changes in central nervous systems. Recently, sex steroids modulations of central nervous systems are mentioned. Progesterone is reported to show anxiolytic and hypnotic activities in rodents. These effects are blocked by a gamma-amino-butyric acid (GABA) A receptor-gated chloride channel antagonist picrotoxin, indicating the $GABA_A$ receptor-mediated action of progesterone. Furthermore, these effects of progesterone are potently blocked by inhibitors of 5α-reductase, the enzyme that converts progesterone into 5α-reduced metabolites (Celotti et al. 1997). The major metabolite of progesterone is 3α-hydroxy-pregnan-20-one (alloprognanolone), a kind of neurosteroids that directly stimulates $GABA_A$ receptor functions (Majewska 1992) and exhibits anxiolytic activity.

Kampo formulations (Japanese traditional herbal medicines) are widely used for the treatment of menopausal syndromes in Japan. In the clinically, Tokishakuyakusan, Kamishoyosan, Keishibukuryogan and Unkeito are widely used. The herbal ingredients of these four Kampo formulations are similar as shown in Fig. 1, however, the clinical uses of these Kampo formulations are different. Therefore we investigate the differences of them from the basic pharmacological and chemical studies.

The purposes of the present study are (1) to evaluate the acute anxiolytic effect of Kampo formulations in mice by using the social interaction test, and (2) to investigate the active component(s) of Kampo formulations.

当帰芍薬散 Tokishakuyakusan	当帰 Angelicae Radix, 芍薬 Paeoniae Radix, 川芎 Cnidii Rhizoma, 沢瀉 Alismatis Rhizoma, 茯苓 Hoelen, 朮 Atractylodis Rhizoma
加味逍遥散 Kamishoyosan	柴胡 Bupleuri Radix, 芍薬 Paeoniae Radix, 朮 Atractylodis Rhizoma, 当帰 Angelicae Radix, 茯苓 Hoelen, 山梔子 Gardeniae Fructus, 牡丹皮 Moutan Cortex, 甘草 Glycyrrhizae Radix, 生姜 Zingiberis Rhizoma, 薄荷 Menthae Herba
桂枝茯苓丸 Keishibukuryogan	桂皮 Cinnamomum Cortex, 茯苓 Hoeren, 牡丹皮 Moutan Cortex, 桃仁 Persicae Semen, 芍薬 Paeoniae Radix
温 経 湯 Unkeito	半夏 Pinelliae Tuber, 麦門冬 Ophiopogonis Tuber, 当帰 Angelica Radix, 川芎 Cnidii Rhizoma, 芍薬 Paeoniae Radix, 人参 Ginseng Radix, 桂皮 Cinnamomum Cortex, 牡丹皮 Moutan Cortex, 甘草 Glycyrrhizae Radix, 呉茱萸 Evodiae Fructus, 生姜 Zingiberis Rhizoma, 阿膠 Asini Corii Collas

Fig.1 Kampo formulations (Japanese traditional herbal medicines)

2 Materials and Methods

Animals: Male ddY mice (Japan SLC, Shizuoka, Japan) were used. Social interaction (SI) tests were performed at the age of 6-7 weeks. The present studies were conducted in accordance with the standards established by the Guide for the Care and Use of Laboratory Animals of Showa University.

Preparation of Kampo formulations: Dried medicinal herbs used for preparation of Kampo formulations. All voucher specimens are on deposit at the herbarium of the School of Pharmacy Showa University. Kampo formulations used in this study were listed in Fig. 1. A single day dose for human adults consists of the formulation mixed with 600 ml of water, and the whole mixture is decocted until the volume is reduced by half. The decoction was freeze-dried to obtain a powder. This powder was dissolved in distilled water just before the experiments,

Social interaction (SI) test: On the day of the SI test, the cages were subjected to the experimental conditions for at least 2 hr. A pair of mice each belonging to a different cage was placed in the test arena (a plastic cage 22 x 15 cm), and the SI behavior between the mice was observed for 5 min. During this period, the cumulative time spent carrying out SI behavior (genital investigation, tail licking, facing, neck licking, and trunk sniffing) was measured (File 1980).

Data analysis: Cumulative SI times over 5 min were represented as means ± S.E. for each group. SI times were statistically analyzed with the

Student's t-test or one-way analysis of variance (ANOVA) followed by Dunnett's test or two-way ANOVA followed by the Student-Newman-Keuls test.

3 Results

Effects of KSS on SI time in mice: When administered orally 1 hr prior to the tests, Kamishoyosan (KSS) and Unkeito increased SI time, but Tokisyakuyakusan and Keishibukuryogan did not have any effect. Although KSS caused dose-dependent increase in SI time, Unkeito was not shown dose dependency. From these results, we focused to study Kamishoyosan (KSS).

Effects of picrotoxin, flumazenil and 5HT$_{1A}$ receptor antagonist on KSS-induced SI behavior: The increase of the SI time by diazepam (3.0 mg/kg) was partly but significantly attenuated by 1 mg/kg picrotoxin, a GABA$_A$ receptor-gated chloride ion channel antagonist (p<0.05) (Fig. 2a). On the other hand, the increase in SI time by KSS (50 mg/kg) was dose-dependently and perfectly antagonized by picrotoxin. To examine the mediation of GABA$_A$/BZP receptors in the anxiolytic action of KSS, the effects of GABA$_A$/BZP receptor antagonist was tested. As shown in Fig. 2b, centrally administered flumazenil, a selective GABA$_A$/BZP receptor antagonist, antagonized the induction of SI behavior by KSS (p<0.01). On

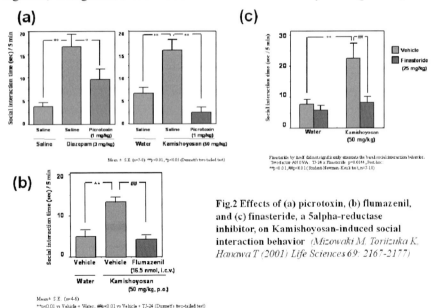

Fig.2 Effects of (a) picrotoxin, (b) flumazenil, and (c) finasteride, a 5alpha-reductase inhibitor, on Kamishoyosan-induced social interaction behavior (Mizowaki M, Toriizuka K, Hanawa T (2001) Life Sciences 69: 2167-2177)

the other hand, intraperitoneal administered NAN-190, a $5HT_{1A}$ receptor antagonist, did not antagonize the induction of SI behavior by KSS.

Effect of finasteride on KSS-induced SI behavior: Acute administration of finasteride (25 mg/kg, -2 hr) in rats is reported to block the conversion of progesterone into allopregnanolone by blocking the enzyme 5α-reductase (Concas et al. 1998). Finasteride itself showed slight but not significant decrease in social interaction time. However, KSS-induced increase ($p<0.01$) was significantly blocked by finasteride to the level of the control ($p<0.05$), indicating that KSS-induced action is mediated by the synthesis of 5α-reduced metabolites (Fig. 2c).

Effects of component herbs in KSS on SI behavior: To clarify the active ingredient in KSS, the effects of the individual component herbs in KSS on SI behavior were examined. An increase of the SI time was observed for hot water extracts of Menthae Herba and Gardeniae Fructus. On the other hand, Solutions of KSS minus one component herb (KSS excluding an individual component herb) were prepared and their activities were measured. When KSS minus Gardeniae Fructus, KSS minus Paeoniae Radix, KSS minus Glycyrrhizae Radix and KSS minus Hoelen were administered to mice, the SI time was significantly reduced to the control level.

Effects of Gardeniae Fructus on the social interaction time: To clarify the active component(s) in Gardeniae Fructus, hot water extract of Gardeniae Fructus was extracted with ethyl alcohol, acetic acid ethyl ester, and water, successively. Finally we determined the active component was geniposide, iridoid glucoside, by spectral analyses. Fig. 3 shows the activity

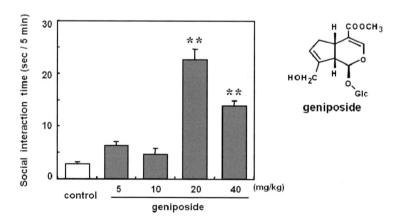

Fig. 3 The effects of geniposide (p.o., n=5) on the cumulative social interaction times for male mice. Geniposide was orally administered 1 hr before the test. Mean ± S.E., *$p<0.05$, **$p<0.01$ vs control (water), one-way ANOVA followed by Dunnett's test. (Toriizuka K, Kamiki H, Ohmura (Yoshikawa) N, et al. (2005) Life Sciences 77: 3010-3020)

of the oral administration of geniposide at a dose of 20 and 40 mg/kg which increased the SI time.

4. Conclusion

In summary, KSS increased SI behavior in mice, indicating that KSS possesses anxiolytic effect. The effect was strongly blocked by $GABA_A$/BZP receptor antagonist, suggesting that KSS-induced effect is mediated by brain $GABA_A$/BZP receptor stimulations. Furthermore, the inhibition of 5α-reductase strongly attenuated the action of KSS, suggesting the possible mediation of neurosteroid synthesis (Mizowaki et al. 2001). And it was revealed that the effects of Gardeniae Fructus and geniposide were related to the pharmacological activities of KSS (Toriizuka et al. 2005). This is the first report of data according to the anxiolytic effects of geniposide, and this newly discovered activity may offer new perspectives for secoiridoid research. Hypothetical model of Kamishoyosan and geniposide action on $GABA_A$ receptor is shown in Fig.4.

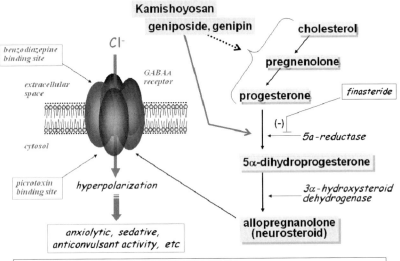

Fig.4 Hypothetical model of Kamishoyosan and geniposide action on $GABA_A$ receptor through the neurosteroids metabolic pathway

Acknowledgements: This work was supported by a Grand-in-Aid for Scientific Research (C) from the Ministry of Education, Science, Sports and Culture, Japan (Grant No. 15590605), and by grants from the Uehara Memorial Foundation (2007).

References

Celotti F, Negri-Cesi P, Poletti A (1997) Steroid metabolism in the mammalian brain, 5α-reduction and aromatization. Brain Res Bull 44: 365-375

Concas A, Mostallino MC, Porcu P, Follesa P, Barbaccia ML, Trabucchi M, Purdy RH, Grisenti A, Biggio G (1998) Role of brain allopregnanolone in the plasticity of gamma-aminobutyric acid type A receptor in rat brain during pregnancy and after delivery. Proc Natl Acad Sci 95: 13284-13289

File SE (1980) The use of social interaction as a method for detecting anxiolytic activity of chlordiazepoxide-like drugs. J Neurosci Methods 2: 219-238

Majewska MD (1992) Neurosteroids, endogenous bimodal modulators of the GABAA receptor. Mechanism of action and physiological significance. Prog Neurobiol 38: 379-395

Mizowaki M, Toriizuka K, Hanawa T (2001) Anxiolytic effect of Kami-Shoyo-San in mice, Possible mediation of neurosteroid synthesis. Life Sciences 69: 2167-2177

Toriizuka K, Kamiki H, Ohmura (Yoshikawa) N, Fujii M, Hori Y, Fukumura M, Hirai Y, Isoda S, Nemoto Y, Ida Y (2005) Anxiolytic effect of Gardeniae Fructus-extract containing active ingredient from Kamishoyosan (KSS), a Japanese traditional Kampo medicine. Life Sciences 77: 3010-3020

Activation of Microglia Induced Learning and Memory Deficits

Sachiko Tanaka[1], Hirokazu Ohtaki[2], Tomoya Nakamachi[2], Satoshi Numazawa[1], Seiji Shioda[2] and Takemi Yoshida[1]

[1]Department of Biochemical Toxicology, Showa University, School of Pharmaceutical Sciences, and [2]Department of Anatomy, Showa University, School of Medicine, 1-5-8 Hatanodai, Shinagawa-ku, Tokyo 142-8555, Japan

stanaka@pharm.showa-u.ac.jp

Summary. We used lipopolysaccharide (LPS) to activate microglia which play an important role in the brain immune system. LPS injected into the rat hippocampus CA1 region activated microglial cells resulting in an increased production of interleukin (IL)-1β and tumor necrosis factor (TNF) α in the hippocampus during the early stage of its treatment. Subacute treatment with LPS for 5 days caused activation of microglia and induced learning and memory deficits in animals when examined with a step-through passive avoidance test. And then we had found the decreased [^{3}H]MK801 binding in the hippocampus CA1, CA3 and DG. The gene expression of NMDA receptor NR1 subunits was also decreased by the LPS treatment. These results suggest that activation of microglia induced by LPS results in a decrease of glutamatergic transmission which leads to learning and memory deficits.

Key words. Lipopolysaccharide, Learning and memory, Microglia, NMDA receptors

1 Introduction

Activation of microglia has been observed during the development of neurodegenerative diseases such as Alzheimer's (AD) and Parkinson's diseases (PD) (McGeer et al., 1998, Dickson et al., 1993). In *in vivo* experiments, activated microglia release inflammatory cytokines such as interleukin (IL)-1β and tumor necrosis factor (TNF) α and also produce oxygen- and nitrogen-centered free radicals that contribute to the neurodegenerative process (Gayle et al., 2002, Jeohn et al., 2000, Wenk et al., 2004). Lipopolysaccharide (LPS) is a bacterial endotoxin known to stimulate the immune system through activation of macrophage-like cells in peripheral tissues (Quann et al., 1994). There are several types of inflammatory animal models using LPS such as Parkinson's diseases, Alzheimer's diseases and white matter diseases. Parkinson's model suggest that LPS injection into the substantia nigra of rats induces loss of TH-immunoreactive neurons (Kim et al., 2000). LPS induces preferential brain white matter injury and affects neurobehavioral performance what occur in most case of white matter diseases (Fan et al., 2005). These animal models seem likely that the activation of microglia contributes to neuronal degeneration. We also developed animal model for learning and memory (Tanaka et al., 2006). LPS injected into the rat hippocampus CA1 region activated microglial cells resulting in an increased production of IL-1β and TNFα in the hippocampus. Subacute treatment with LPS for 5 days induced learning and memory deficits in animals when examined with a step-through passive avoidance test, but histochemical analysis revealed that neuronal cell death was not observed under these experimental conditions. This model also showed that inflammation can be a trigger for changing a neuronal function. It is still obscure how activated microglia affect the development and survival of neuronal cells and modulate neuronal functions. Willard et al. (2000) have reported that cytotoxicity due to the chronic neuroinflammation evoked by LPS can be rescued by the NMDA antagonist mematine or the COX2 inhibitor CI987. Glutamate transmission, especially via NMDA receptors, is very important in facets of memory function such as the induction of LTP (Malgaroli and Tsien 1992, Bliss and Collingridge, 1993). Therefore, it is required to determine whether there are any changes in NMDA receptors in our model animal.

2 Methods

2.1 Surgery and drug treatment

All animal experiments were conducted under the Showa University Animal Experiment and Welfare Regulations. Male Wistar rats were anesthetized with sodium pentobarbital (50 mg/kg, i.p.) and immobilized in a stereotaxic flame to implant a guide cannula for injection of LPS into the hippocampal CA1 region (3.5 mm posterior, 2.2 mm lateral, and 4.3 mm ventral from the bregma) and fixed to the skull with dental cement. Rats were injected with LPS (20 µg) dissolved in 2 µl of phosphate buffered saline (PBS) or PBS alone under diethyl ether anesthesia.

Subacute treatment with LPS (20 μg/day) was performed for 5 consecutive days.

2.2 Passive Avoidance Procedure

Passive avoidance test was carried out at 2 hr after final LPS injection. In the acquisition trial, each rat was placed in the lighted compartment and allowed to enter the dark compartment through the guillotine door. Once the rat entered the dark compartment, foot shock was immediately delivered. The number of foot shocks required to retain the animal in the lighted compartment for 3 min was recorded as a measure of the acquisition of passive avoidance. The second session was carried out 24 h after the first session. The rat was placed in the lighted compartment and the retention latency, the time elapsed before the time when the rat stepped through to the dark compartment, was recorded as a measure of the retention of passive avoidance. If the rat did not step through the dark compartment within 300 seconds, a ceiling score of 300 seconds was assigned.

2.3 Immunohistochemistry

Rats were sacrificed at 6 hr after final LPS injection for 5 days, and their hippocampi were removed. For CD11b immunostaining, sections were preincubated in 2.5% normal horse serum after endogeneuos peroxidase blocking by 0.3% H_2O_2 and incubated with monoclonal mouse anti-rat CD11b antibody (1:1000). Sections were rinsed and incubated with biotinylated horse anti-mouse IgG (1:200, VECTASTAIN ABC kit, Vector, Burlingame, CA) and then incubated in an avidin-biotin complex solution followed by diaminobenzidine (DAB kit, Vector).

2.4 [^{3}H]MK-801 binding

[^{3}H]MK-801 binding was measured by the method previously described (Tanaka et al., 1997). Tissue sections on slides were thawed at room temperature and preincubated in 50 mM Tris-HCl buffer (pH 7.4) for 1 hr. Sections were dried with cold air and then incubated for 2 hr at room temperature in 50 mM Tris-HCl buffer containing 10 nM [^{3}H]MK-801. Non-specific binding was measured in the presence of 10 mM cold MK-801 and represented less than 5% of total binding. After incubation, sections were rinsed twice for 2 min, twice for 40 min in ice-cold buffer, once for 1 min in ice-cold water, and then dried under a stream of cold air. Radioactivities in autoradiograms were quantitatively determined with an image analyzer (Fujix Bas3000, Fuji Photo Film Co., Tokyo, Japan).

2.5 Gene expression

Total RNA was extracted using the QIAGEN RNeasy Lipid Tissue Mini kit (QIAGEN, Hilden, Germany). Real time RT-PCR was carried out by QuantiTect SYBR Green RT-PCR (QIAGEN). Primers for NR1, NR2A and GAPDH were prepared by QuantiTect Primer Assays (QIAGEN).

2.6 Statistical analysis

Statistical analysis between PBS-treated and LPS-treated group was performed with the Mann-Whitney test.

3 Results

3.1 LPS induces activation of microglia and impairment of learning and memory in rats

An experiment was conducted to determine whether microglia were activated by LPS treatment or not. We demonstrated the long-term activation of microglia after subacute treatment with LPS for 5 days (Fig. 1). CD11b immunopositive cells increased in the subacute LPS-treated group as compared with the PBS-treated group. We also determined the increased IL-1β and TNFα using ELISA methods. In the PBS-treated rats, the contents of IL-1β and TNFα were very low. IL-1β and TNFα contents significantly increased up to 622pg/mg and 174 pg/me protein, respectively, at 2 hr after LPS injection.

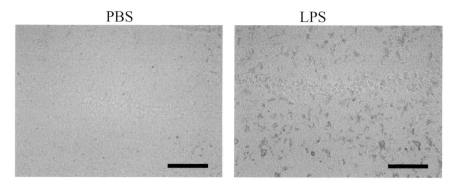

Fig. 1. Immunohistochemical analysis of the effect of subacute LPS treatment on CD11b-positive microglia in the hippocampus. LPS (20 μg/2 μL/injection) or PBS (2 μL/injection) injected into the hippocampus CA1 area for 5 consecutive days. Representative photomicrographs are coronal sections of the CA1 field of the hippocampus at 6 hr after the final LPS injection, 6 hr after the final PBS injection. Scare bars = 100 μm

The performance abilities in the passive avoidance task of rats treated with PBS or LPS (20 µg/2 µl/day) for 5 days are summarized in Table 1. LPS treatment significantly increased the number of electric shocks needed for acquisition of passive avoidance. Retention latency from light to dark was significantly reduced by LPS treatment. Furthermore, locomotions for 5 min were recorded to clarify whether learning and memory deficits were related to differences in locomotor activity or not; there was no significant difference between the PBS- and LPS-treated groups in locomotor activity (data not shown). These results indicate that LPS treatment for 5 consecutive days caused learning and memory deficits.

Table 1. Effect of LPS treatment on rat performance in the passive avoidance test.

Treatment	Number of foot shocks	Retention latency (s)
PBS-treated (n= 6)	1.3 ± 0.2	290.0 ± 10.0
LPS-treated (n= 6)	2.5 ± 0.3*	141.3 ± 46.2*

LPS (20 µg/2 µL/ injection) was injected into the hippocampus CA1 area daily for 5 consecutive days. The acquisition trail was conducted 1 hr after PBS or LPS treatment. The number of foot shocks required to retain the rats on the safe compartment for 3 min was recorded as an index of acquisition of passive avoidance, and retention latency was determined 24 hr after the acquisition trial as an index of retention of passive avoidance. Results are presented as the mean ± SE. *$p<0.05$ compared with the PBS-treated group.

3.2 Changes of NMDA receptors after subacute treatment with LPS

[^{3}H]MK-801 bindings were highest in strarum radiatum and stratum oriens of the hippocampus CA1 area followed by those in CA2 and CA3. Quantitative analysis of [^{3}H]MK-801 bindings performed with an image analyzer on the CA1, CA3, DG and cortex area. Specific [^{3}H]MK-801 bindings in LPS-treated rats were significantly attenuated to 78, 86, 75% of that seen in CA1, CA2, and DG of the PBS-treated rats. The gene expression levels of these receptors were examined in PBS- and LPS-treated group. LPS treatment for 5 days resulted in a significant decrease in the NR1 subunits of NMDA receptors.

4 Discussion

In this study, we found activation of microglia after subacute treatment with LPS for 5 days (Fig. 1). Immunoreactivity for CD11b in the tissue section from rats treated with PBS was rare and only weakly expressed in the injected area. CD11b immunopositive cells increased in the subacute LPS-treated group. In our previous study, to identify the cells expressing IL-1β after LPS treatment, a double-labeled immunohistochemical study was performed between IL-1β and two of the cell markers, CD11b and GFAP (Tanaka et al., 2006). After LPS treatment, IL-1β immunopositive cells increased and then co-localized with those for CD11b, but not GFAP. These results suggest that LPS treatment caused an increase of both IL-1β expression and IL-1β immunopositive cells which were indicative of microglia.

Glutamate transmission, especially via NMDA receptors, has been shown to be very important in facets of memory function such as the induction of LTP (Malgaroli and Tsien 1992, Bliss and Collingridge, 1993). NMDA receptors are heteromeric complexes containing both NR1 and NR2 subunits (Cull-Candy et al., 2001). We found the decrease of [^{3}H]MK-801 binding and gene expression of NR1 subunit in the hippocampus after subacute LPS treatment. These data show that glutamatergic transmission was attenuated in LPS-treated rats.

The findings presented herein provide evidence that activation of microglia induced by LPS causes functional change in the hippocampus such as attenuated glutamatergic transmission which leads to learning and memory deficits.

Acknowledgments

This work was supported in part by a Showa University Grant-in Aid for Innovative Collaborative Research Projects.

References

Bliss TV, Collongridge GL (1993) A synaptic model of memory: long-term potentiation in the hippocampus. Nature 361: 31-39

Cull-Candy S, Brickley S, Farrant M (2001) NMDA receptor subunits: diversity, development and disease. Curr Opin Neurobiol, 11: 327-335

Dickson DW, Lee SC, Mattiace LA, Yen SH, Brosnan C (1993) Microglia and cytokines in neurological disease, with special reference to AIDS and Alzheimer's disease. Glia 7: 78-83

Fan LW, Pang Y, Lin S, Rhodes PG, Cai Z (2005) Minocycline attenuates lipopolysaccharide-induced white matter injury in the neonatal rat brain. Neurosci 133: 159-168

Gayle D, Ling Z, Tong C, Landers T, Lipton JW, Carvey PM (2002) Lipopolysaccharide (LPS)-induced dopamine cell loss in culture: roles of tumor necrosis factor-alpha, interleukin-1beta, and nitric oxide. Brain Res Dev Brain Res 133: 27-35

Jeohn GH, Kim WG, Hong JS (2000) Time dependency of the action of nitric oxide in lipopolysaccharide-interferon-gamma-induced neuronal cell death in murine primary neron-glia co-cultures. Brain Res 880: 173-177

Kim WG, Mohney RP, Wilson B, Jeohn GH, Liu B, Hong JS (2000) Regional difference in susceptibility to lipopolysaccharide-induced neurotoxicity in the rat brain: role of microglia. J Neurosci 20: 6309-6316

Malgaroli A, Tsien RW (1992) Glutamate-induced long term potentiation of the frequency of miniature synaptic currents in cultured hippocampal neurons. Nature 357: 134-139

McGeer PL, Itagaki S, Boyes BE, McGeer EG (1998) Reactive microglia are positive for HLA-DR in the substantia nigra of Parkinson's and Alzheimer's disease brains. Neurol 38: 1285-1291

Quan N, Sundar SK, Weiss JM (1994) Induction of interleukin-1 in various brain regions after peripheral and central injections of lipopolysaccharide. J Neuroimmunol 49: 125-134

Tanaka S, Kiuchi Y, Numazawa S, Oguchi K, Yoshida T, Kuroiwa Y (1997) Changes in glutamate receptors, c-fos mRNA expression and activator protein-1 (AP-1) DNA binding activity in the brain of phenobarbital-dependent and withdrawn rats. Brain Res 756: 35-45

Tanaka S, Ide M, Shibutani T, Ohtaki H, Numazawa S, Shioda S, Yoshida T (2006) Lipopolysaccharide-induced microglial activation induces learning and memory deficits without neuronal cell death in rats. J Neurosci Res 83: 557-566

Wenk G, McGann K, Hauss-Wegrzyniak B, Ronchetti D. Maucci R., Rosi S., Gasparini L, Ongini E (2004) Attenuation of chronic neuroinflammtion by a nitric oxide0releasing derivative of the antioxidant ferulic acid. J Neurochem 89: 484-493

Willard L, Hauss-Wegrzyniak B, Danysz W, Wenk G (2000) The toxicity of chronic neuroinflammtion upon basal forebrain cholinergic neurons of rats can be attenuated by glutamatergic antagonism or cyclooxygenase-2. Exp Brain Res 134: 58-65

Increased behavioral activity with regular circadian rhythm in PACAP specific receptor (PAC1) transgenic mice

Satoru Arata[1], Tomohiko Hosono[1], Yoshitaka Taketomi[1], Haruaki Kageyama[2], Tomoya Nakamachi[2], Seiji Shioda[2]

[1]Center for Biotechnology, Showa University, Hatanodai, Shinagawa-ku, Tokyo 142-8555, Japan
 <e-mail> arata@pharm.showa-u.ac.jp, thosono@med.showa-u.ac.jp, takedomi@pharm.showa-u.ac.jp
[2]Department of Anatomy, Showa University School of Medicine, 1-5-8 Hatanotai, Shinagawa-ku, Tokyo 142-8555, Japan
<e-mail> haruaki@med.showa-u.ac.jp, nakamachi@med.showa-u.ac.jp, shioda@med.showa-u.ac.jp

Summary. To define the physiological roles of Pituitary adenylate cyclase-activating polypeptide (PACAP), we developed PACAP specific receptor (PAC1) transgenic (Tg) mice using the Cre/loxP recombination system. wPAC1 Tg mice, which express the *Pac1* transgene in their entire body, showed increased behavioral activity in the dark period of a 12-h light/dark cycle (Zeitegeber time 0 (ZT0) = lights on, ZT12= lights off). LNL-PAC1/CaMKII-Cre double Tg mice (hPAC1 Tg mice), which undergo Cre/loxP recombination in hippocampal nerve cells, expressed the *Pac1* transgene in the hippocampus. hPAC1 Tg mice showed increased behavioral activity (150% or more compared to control) in the early dark period (ZT 12-17), which is the most active time for wild type mice. However, there was no change in circadian rhythm. Similar hyperactivity was observed in LNL-PAC1/CaMKII-CreER double Tg mice (ihPAC1 Tg mice) when the mice were treated with tamoxifen to induce Cre/loxp recombination in adulthood. Moreover, immunohistochemical analysis of LNL-PAC1/LNL-Venus/ CaMKII-CreER triple Tg mice treated with tamoxifen, revealed that PAC1 transgene were expressed in hippocampal nerve cells. These results suggest that the expression of the *PAC1* transgene, especially in hippocampal nerve cells, may enhance the behavioral activity associated with regular circadian rhythm.

Key Words. PAC1 receptor, transgenic mice, locomotor activity

1. Introduction

Pituitary adenylate cyclase-activating polypeptide (PACAP) is a highly conserved neuropeptide that plays important roles in the development of the nervous system and the maintenance of homeostasis (Shioda, 2006). PACAP specific receptor (PAC1) is a G-protein-coupled receptor that binds PACAP with a thousandfold higher affinity than the related peptide VIP (vasoactive intestinal peptide). PAC1 is widely distributed in the central nervous system and in peripheral tissue (Shivers et al., 1991). PAC-1-mediated signaling has been implicated in a variety of biological processes, such as neurotropic actions, pituitary function, circadian rhythms, and learning and memory. Thus, PACAP signals are essential for ontogeny and physiological functions. It has been reported that both PACAP deficient mice and PAC-1 deficient mice have a high rate of mortality by two weeks after birth (Hashimoto et al., 2001; Otto et al., 2004). However, the mechanism of this fatal congenital abnormality is not clear. To assess the function of PACAP signaling *in vivo*, we generated PAC1 transgenic (Tg) mice using the Cre/loxP recombination system.

2. Generation of PAC1 transgenic mice

To construct the Cre-mediated *PAC1* transgene, the PAC1 cDNA was inserted into the EcoR1 site of the pCALNL5 vector (Kanegae et al., 1996) and excised with the HindIII and SalI sites to produce a *CAG* promotor-loxP-neo^r-loxP-PAC1 (LNL-PAC1) fragment. The purified fragment was microinjected into C57BL/6 fertilized eggs, and LNL-PAC1 Tg mice were generated by standard methods. For the expression of the *PAC1* transgene in the entire body, LNL-PAC1 Tg mice were mated with Pgk2-Cre Tg mice, in which the *Cre* transgene is controlled by the spermatogenic cell-specific promoter of *pgk2* (Kido et al., 2005). F1 male mice with germline transmission of both transgenes were bred with C57BL/6 female mice. The F2 offspring that harbored the PAC1 transgene, which contained an excised floxed neo^r transgene, were named whole body-PAC1 (wPAC1) Tg mice. For hippocampus-specific expression of the PAC1 transgene, we generated CaMKII-Cre Tg mice using the α subunit of calcium-calmodulin-dependent protein kinase II (CaMKII) promoter and Cre transgene, and CaMKII-CreER Tg mice using the CaMKII promoter and the Cre-estrogen-like receptor fusion (CreER) transgene. LNL-PAC1 Tg mice were mated with CaMKII-Cre Tg mice or CaMKII-CreER Tg mice. The resulting F1 offspring, which harbored the LNL-PAC1/CaMKII-Cre double transgenes or the LNL-PAC1/CaMKII-CreER double transgenes, were named hippocampus PAC1 (hPAC1)-Tg mice or tamoxifen-induced hippocampus PAC1 (ihPAC1) Tg mice, respectively. All mice were housed with a 12-h light/dark cycle with ad libitum access to food and water. The experimental protocol was approved by The Institutional Animal Care and Use Committee of Showa University.

3. Expression of PAC1 transgene

PAC1 mRNA was detected by RT-PCR in several tissues of the wPAC1 Tg mice such as heart, liver, kidney and brain, while low levels of endogenous *PAC1* mRNA were only detected in the brain and testis of wild-type mice.

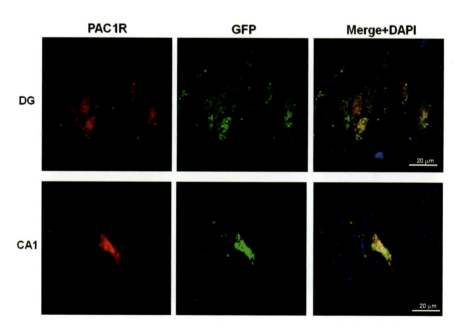

Fig. 1. Tamoxifen induced PAC1 expression in the hippocampus of ihPAC1 Tg mice. Fluorescent images showing immunostaining of the dentate gyrus (DG) and CA1 region of the hippocampus of LNL-PAC1/LNL-Venus/CaMKII-Cre triple Tg mice after tamoxifen treatment. GFP-like and PAC1-like immunoreactivity were co-localized.

Moreover, both hPAC1 Tg mice and tamoxifen-treated ihPAC1 Tg mice expressed the transgenic *PAC1* mRNA in brain, but not other tissues. Immunohistochemical analysis of LNL-PAC1/LNL-Venus/CaMKII-CreER triple Tg mice treated with tamoxifen, revealed that PAC1 and Venus a variant of green fluorescent protein (GFP) were expressed in several dentate gyrus cells and some CA1 cells, and that the gene products were co-localized (Fig. 1). These results suggest that our PAC1 Tg mice with conditional expression of PAC1 are functioning as planned.

4. Behavioral activity of PAC1 Tg mice

To assess the behavior of PAC1 Tg mice, we examined spontaneous locomotor activity in each animal's home cage using an ACTIO-100 unit (EIKOU Science). The early dark period (ZT12-17) is the most active time for wild type C57BL/6 mice. The locomotor activity of wPAC1 Tg mice increased in dark periods as compared with littermate wild type mice (Fig. 2a). Furthermore, hPAC1 Tg mice clearly showed increased locomotor activity in the early dark period (ZT12-17). The locomotor activity of hPAC1 Tg mice was 150% that of control littermate mice. Increased behavioral activity was also observed in aged hPAC1 Tg mice, while the activity of littermate control was reduced (Fig. 2b-d). However, the amount of food and water consumed and circadian rhymes were unchanged.

Similar hyperactivity in the dark period was observed in ihPAC1 Tg mice after tamoxifen treatment in adulthood. These results suggest that PAC1 expression in the hippocampus increases the behavioral activity, and that induction of PAC1 in adulthood has a similar effect.

5. Discussions

This study demonstrates behavioral hyperactivity with regular circadian rhythm in PAC1 transgenic mice. The remarkable increase of locomotor activity in hPAC1 Tg mice was seen in the early dark period (ZT12-17), which is the most active time for wild type mice, but not in the light period(ZT 0-11), which is an inactive time. Although spontaneous locomotor activity was decreased in aged wild type mice, an increase in spontaneous locomotor activity was observed in aged hPAC1 Tg mice. Furthermore, this increase in activity was also seen when PAC1 expression was induced in adulthood. These results suggest that PAC1 plays important roles in behavioral hyperactivity.

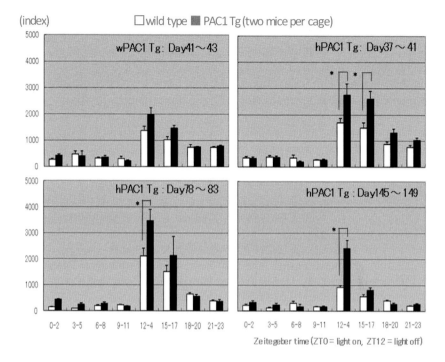

Fig. 2. Increased behavioral activity of wPAC1 Tg mice (a) and hPAC1 Tg mice (b-d). The locomotor activities of PAC1 Tg mice were examined for 3-5 days in a 12-h light/dark cycle (Zeitegeber time 0 (ZT0) = lights on, ZT12 = lights off) at the indicated ages. The number of times that each mouse crossed the infrared sensor (2-cm interval) in each time zone was expressed. *, p<0.05 *versus* wild type.

PACAP is a potent stimulator of cAMP accumulation in the rodent central nervous system, and evidence suggests that PACAP is an endogenous psychostimulant (Arimura, 1992; Masuo et al., 2004). Central administration of PACAP in adult rats causes behavioral hyperactivity and hypothermia (Masuo et al., 1995). PACAP is also expressed in the hypothalamic suprachiasmatic nucleus (SCN), which regulates circadian rhythms. PACAP is co-expressed with glutamate, an essential modulator of light entrainment (Hannibal et al., 2000). It was also reported that, similar to light, PACAP can phase shift the endogenous rhythm (Harrington et al., 1999; Nielson et al., 2001). Moreover, Hannibal has reported that light stimulation in the early night resulted in larger phase delays in PAC1 deficient mice compared with wild-type mice, and that this was accompanied by a marked reduction in light-induced *mPer1*, *mPer2*, and *c-fos* gene expression. These observations indicate that PAC1 signaling participates in the gating control of photic sensitivity of the clock (Hannibal et al., 2001).

Our results from this PAC1 Tg mice study are not contradictory to current knowledge. The induction of PAC1 in brain may be useful for the improvement of locomotor behavior with regular circadian rhythms.

References

Arimura A (1992) Receptors for pituitary adenylate cyclase-activating polypeptide: comparison with vasoactive intestinal peptide receptors, Trends Endocrinol Metab 3:288-294

Otto C, Hein L, Brede M, Jahns R, Engelhardt S, Grone HJ, Schutz, G (2004) Pulmonary hypertension and right heart failure in pituitary adenylate cyclase-activating cyclase-activating polypeptide type 1 receptor-deficient mice. Circulation 110:3245-3251

Hannibal J, Moller M, Ottersen OP, Fahrenkrug J (2000) PACAP and glutamate are co-stored in the retinohypothalamic tract. J Comp Neurol 418:147-155

Hannibal J, Francoise J, Harriette Nielsen HS, Laurant J, Brabet P, Fahrenkrug J (2001) Dissociation between light-induced phase shift on the circadian rhythm and clock gene expression in mice lacking the pituitary adenylate cyclase activating polypeptide type 1 receptor. J Neuroscience 21:4883-4890

Harrington ME, Hoque S, Hall A, Golombek D, Biello S (1999) Pituitary adenylate cyclase- activating peptide phase shifts circadian rhythms in a manner similar to light. J Neurol. 19:6637-6642

Hashimoto H, Shintani N, Tanaka K, Mori W, Hirose M., Matsuda T., Sakaue M, Miyazaki J, Niwa H, Tashiro F, Yamamoto K, Koga K, Tomimoto S, Kunugi A, Suetake S, Baba A (2001) Altered psychomotor behaviors in mice lacking pituitary adenylate cyclase-activating cyclase-activating polypeptide (PACAP). Proc Natl Acad Sci U.S.A. 98:13355-13360

Kanegae Y, Takamori K, Sato Y, Lee G, Nakai M, Saito I (1996) Efficient gene activation system on mammalian cell chromosomes using recombinant adenovirus producing Cre recombinase. Gene 181:207-212

Kido T, Arata S, Suzuki R, Hosono T, Nakanishi Y, Miyazaki J, Saito I, Kuroki T, Shioda S (2005) The testicular fatty acid binding protein PERF15 regulates the fate of germ cells in PERF15 transgenic mice. Dev Growth Differ. 47:15-24

Masuo Y, Noguchi J, Morita S, Matsumoto Y (1995) Effects of intracerebroventricular administration of pituitary adenylate cyclase-activating polypeptide (PACAP) on the motor activity and reserpine-induced hypothermia in murines. Brain Res. 700:219-226

Masuo Y, Morita M, Oka S, Ishido M (2004) Motor hyperactivity caused by a deficit in dopaminergic neurons and the effects of endocrine disruptor: study inspired by the physiological roles of PACAP in the brain. Regul Pept 123:225-234

Nielsen HS, Hannibal J, Knudsen SM, Fahrenkrug J (2001) Pituitary adenylate cyclase-activating polypeptide induces Period1 and Period2 gene expression in the rat suprachiasmstic nucleus during late night. Neuroscience 103:433-441

Shioda S, Ohtaki H, Nakamachi T, Dohi K, Watanabe J, Nakajo S, Arata S, Kitamura S, Okuda H, Takenoya F, Kitamura Y (2006) Pleiotropic functions of PACAP in the CNS: neuroprotection and neurodevelopment. Ann N Y Acad Sci., 1070:550-60

Shivers BD, Gorce TJ, Gottschall, PE, Arimura, A (1991) Two high affinity binding sites for pituitary adenylate cyclase activating polypeptide have different tissue distribution. Endocrinology 128:3055-3065

Expression and localization of pituitary adenylate cyclase-activating polypeptide (PACAP) specific receptor (PAC1R) after traumatic brain injury in mice

Kentaro Morikawa[1], Kenji Dohi[1], Sachiko Yofu[2], Yuko Mihara[1], Tomoya Nakamachi[2], Hirokazu Ohtaki[2], Seiji Shioda[2] and Tohru Aruga[1]

[1]Department of Emergency and Critical Care Medicine, [2]Department of Anatomy, Showa University School of Medicine, 1-5-8 Hatanodai, Shinagawa-ku, Tokyo, 142-8555 Japan <e-mail> kdop@med.showa-u.ac.jp

Summary. PACAP is a pleiotropic peptide and is well known to suppress neuronal cell death after ischemic injury through PACAP specific receptor (PAC1R). However, the pathological role of PAC1R is not elicited well on traumatic injured brain. Therefore, the purpose of this study is to investigate the expression and localization of PAC1R after traumatic brain injury (TBI) with immunohistochemistry. The PAC1R-immunoreactions (ir) were detected in peri-contusional area 3h after TBI and gradually increased up to 7d. Double immunohistochemical studies were revealed that the PAC1R-ir were co-localized with a microglial marker, CD11b. At 7d after TBI, the PAC1R-ir were merged with CD11b and with GFAP, an astroglial marker. These results suggested that PAC1R expresses in microglia and astrocyte with different time points after TBI, and PACAP and its receptor might play an important role for brain injury as well as ischemia.

Key words. PACAP, traumatic brain injury (TBI), controlled cortical impact (CCI), glial cells

1 Introduction

Traumatic brain injury (TBI) is a critical condition in the field of emergency medicine. In the westernized countries such as the United States and Japan, acute trauma death is the third major cause of death.

PACAP is a pleiotropic neuropeptide and belongs to the secretin/ glucagon/ vasoactive intestinal peptide (VIP) family. Several in vivo and in vitro studies have indicated that PACAP prevented neuronal cell death. PACAP binds to three receptors, two VIP/PACAP receptors (VPAC1R and VPAC2R) and PACAP specific receptor (PAC1R), which are seven transmembrane G protein-coupled receptors. PACAP can bind to PAC1R 1000-times higher affinity and it has been considering that PACAP prevents the neuronal cell death mediated by PAC1R (Arimura 1998). So far, it has been reported that the PAC1R is actively expressed in different neuroepithelia from early developmental stages and expressed in various brain regions during prenatal and postnatal development. However, it still remains as a controversial the role of PACAP and PAC1R on brain injury. In this study, we investigated the expression and localization of PAC1R after TBI of mice in a time-dependent manner.

2 Materials and Methods

Adult male C57/BL6 mice (Saitama, Saitama, Japan) were anesthetized with sodium pentobarbital (50mg/kg, ip).The animals were fixed on a stereotaxic frame and made carefully a burr hole on the left parietal bone with dental drill. Then, the animals were subjected to TBI by controlled cortical impact (a velocity of 5.82 m/s, duration of 47 ms, depth of 1.2 mm, and with a driving pressure of 73 psi) using an electrical compression device adapted for mice (eCCI Model 6.3; Custom Design, Richmond, VA). After injury, the mice perfused with saline followed by 2% PFA during 7 days, and prepared frozen blocks. All procedures involving animals were approved by The Institutional Animal Care and Use Committee of Showa University.

After immersed in H_2O_2, and treated with 10% normal goat serum (NGS), cryosections (8-μm) were then incubated in rabbit anti-PAC1R antibody (1:400, Suzuki et al. 2003) and were detected with biotinylated goat anti-rabbit IgG (1:200, Vector, Burlingame, CA) followed by ABC/DAB (Vector).

For double-staining, the sections (3 to 4 mice brains) were incubated with anti-PAC1R antibody (1:400) and any following primary antibody: mouse anti-GFAP (1:1000, Sigma, St Louis, MO); rat anti-CD11b (1:500, Serotec, Oxford, UK); mouse anti-NeuN (1:400, Chemicon, Temecula, CA) and detected using Alexa fluoresence-labeled secondary antibodies followed by DAPI (1:10,000, Roche, Manheim, Germany).

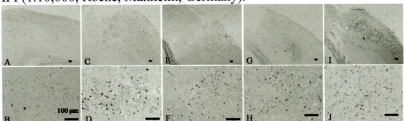

Fig. 1. Representative images of the PAC1R immunoreactions at 0 hour (A, B), 3 hour (C, D), 1 day (E, F), 4 days (G, H) or 7 days (I, J) after TBI. The PAC1R-ir was detected clearly in the perifocal area of the lesions at 3 hours after injury and expressed continuously during experimental periods. Scale bars = 100 μm.

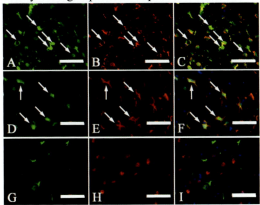

Fig. 2. PAC1R expressing cells 7d after TBI. PAC1R antibody (*green*) was co-stained with antibodies for CD11b (A–C), GFAP (D–F), or Neu N (G–I), respectively (*red*). Arrows are merged cells. Blue in C, F and I is DAPI nuclear staining. Scale bars = 50 μm.

3 Results and Discussion

PAC1R immunoreactions (ir) were detected in the perifocal area of the lesions from 3h after TBI (Fig. 1), and the intensity and number gradually increased up to 7d. PAC1R-expressing cells were identified at 1 and 7d in the perifocal area after TBI. Labelling with microglial (CD11b), astrtoglial (GFAP) or neuronal (NeuN) marker, the PAC1R-ir were merged with CD11b (+) cells, meaning microglia at 1d but no astrocytes and neurons were merged (data not shown). On the 7d, PAC1R-ir were co-localized with microglia and astrocytes, but not or less with neurons (Fig. 2).

In the present study, PAC1R was increased after TBI and expressed in the microglia and astrocytes with different time point. PAC1R-ir were observed in the reactive astrocytes at 5d after a stab wound but not at 2d post surgery (Suzuki et al, 2003). We have also reported PAC1R expressed in neurons (Ohtaki et al, 2008). The diversity of PAC1R expressions could not explain only the differences of animal species. The PAC1R expressions might be different by the pathophysiological features of models such as inflammation and/or apoptosis. Further experiments will be needed to clarify these points. PACAP prevents post-ischemic neuronal cell death after ischemia. PACAP injection decreased hippocampus neuronal death along with an increase of interleukin-6 and inhibition of JNK and p38 phosphorylation after global ischemia (Dohi et al, 2002). Endogenous PACAP also played a critical role in the prevention of neuronal death after focal ischemia. PACAP decreased cytochrome c release from mitochondria by means of the regulation of bcl-2 (Ohtaki et al, 2008). The new insight of PAC1R expression and localization after TBI would contribute understanding for neuroprotective mechanisms of PACAP in brain pathology.

Acknowledgement

This study was supported by the Japanese Ministry of Education, Science, Sports and Culture to K. D. (18591989), a Showa University Grant-in Aid for Innovative Collaborative Research Projects, and a Special Research Grant-in Aid for Development of Characteristic Education from the Japanese Ministry of Education, Culture, Sports, Science and Technology.

References

Arimura A (1998) Perspectives on pituitary adenylate cyclase activating polypeptide (PACAP) in the neuroendocrine, endocrine, and nervous systems. Jpn J Physiol 48:301 – 331

Dohi K, Mizushima H, Nakajo S, Ohtaki H, Matsunaga S, Aruga T, Shioda S (2002) Pituitary adenylate cyclase-activating polypeptide (PACAP) prevents hippocampal neurons from apoptosis by inhibiting JNK/SAPK and p38 signal transduction pathways. Regul Pept 109:83 – 88

Ohtaki H, Nakamachi T, Dohi K, Shioda S. (2008) Role of PACAP in Ischemic Neural Death. J Mol Neurosci 36:16-25

Suzuki R, Arata S, Nakajo S, Ikenaka K, Kikuyama S, Shioda S (2003) Expression of the receptor for pituitary adenylate cyclase-activating polypeptide (PAC1-R) in reactive astrocytes. Brain Res Mol Brain Res 115:10-20

Key Word Index

A
adaptation   125
airway resistance   115
antiopiate   3
anxiety   52
anxiolytic   184
autism   83, 90

B
behavioural tests   52

C
calcium   156
catecholamine   83
concepts   3
controlled cortical impact (CCI)   207
Cre-loxP system   175

D
dipole tracing method   125, 138
double-chamber plethysmograph   115

E
EEG   125, 138
emotion   161

F
facial expression   161
feeding   32
fetal brain   83

G
gardeniae fructus   184
gene therapy   19
glial cells   207
green fluorescent protein   42

H
5-HT   83, 115
hypoglossal nucleus   115
hypothalamus   19, 32, 42

K
Kampo medicines   184

L
learning and memory   191
life-span   19
limb bud mesenchyme   175
limbic system   125
lipopolysaccharide   191
locomotor activity   199

M
melodic intonation therapy   103
mental depression   3
mesencephalic trigeminal sensory neuron   179
metabolic syndrome   19
microdialysis   115
microglia   191
MIF-1   3
MNI   138
MRI   90
MSH   3
music therapy   103
myotonic dystrophy type 1   161

N
neuroimaging   90
neuronal network   32
neuropeptide   42
neuropeptide W (NPW)   32
neuropeptide Y   52
neurorehabilitation   103

neurosteroid   184
nitric oxide   156
NMDA receptors   191

O
obesity   19
olfaction   125
ontogeny   52
orexin   179

P
PAC1 receptor   199
PACAP   207
Parkinson's disease   3
peptide   3
pre-SMA   138
putamen   138

R
Rac1   175
rat   32, 179
recovery   103
respiration   125
ryanodine receptor   156

S
sedation   52
sex difference   90
singing   103
skeleton   19
social brain   90
social cognition   161
social interaction test   184
stroke   103

T
tDCS   103
transcranial direct current stimulation   103
transgenic mice   42, 199
traumatic brain injury (TBI)   207

V
valproate   83

W
whole cell patch-clamp recording   179